FASTer Way to Fat Loss

AMANDA TRESS

FASTer Way to Fat Loss
Non-Fiction

Cover designed by Danielle Sauvageau
Ebook productions by E-books Done Right at www.ebooksdoneright.com
Typesetting by Kelly Jopson-Brown

Visit www.FASTerwaytofatloss.com for more information about the author, updates, or new books.

ISBN
9781098797164

Table of Contents

TO MY BEST FRIEND BRANDON,
AND MY DEEPEST LOVES, EMMA, COLE, AND LILY.
YOU ARE MY *WHY*.

TO MY FASTER WAY COACHES, CLIENTS, AND INFLUENCERS --
THANK YOU FOR YOUR ONGOING ENTHUSIASM
AND SUPPORT FOR THE FASTER WAY.
I AM FOREVER GRATEFUL.

Note from the Author

A big thank you for purchasing the FASTer Way to Fat Loss book! I cannot wait to take you on an incredible journey that will potentially transform your life and empower you to feel healthier than ever.

As a personal trainer and fitness professional, it is incredibly important to me that you remember that not every diet and exercise plan is right for every person. So much is dependent upon your medical history and risk factors. Before making any changes to your diet or exercise plan, please discuss with your physician whether or not the FASTer Way to Fat Loss is right for you.

Additionally, we cannot guarantee that you will see any specific results from the FASTer Way to Fat Loss. Your individual results may vary.

I WISH YOU GREAT SUCCESS IN YOUR JOURNEY.

The FASTer Way to Fat Loss
Introduction

I distinctly remember sitting in my doctor's office as a teenager and hearing him say, "Amanda, you'll be on blood pressure medication for the rest of your life."

That's something that many of us would expect to hear when we're in our seventies. I was seventeen.

He drew me a prison and said I couldn't get out . . . without once asking about my lifestyle. He never asked me what I was eating on a regular basis or if I was exercising consistently. He just said, "Here's a prescription for the rest of your life."

At the time, I was going through a lot! Being student body president, captain of the volleyball and soccer teams, and a senior in high school meant a busy life, so adding heart palpitations, insomnia, and the threat of pills to control my blood pressure was the last thing I wanted.

Because of my busy schedule, I ate fast food any chance I could get. In fact, my favorite meals consisted of burgers, fries, Italian ice, and custard after sports games. There was even a running joke amongst my friends and their dad's that I had a hollow leg. Let's be clear—I could EAT!

By that time, my family had tried many diets—including a bacon and grapefruit diet, which isn't as fun as it sounds. The diets did little to encourage a healthy lifestyle at home, and my sisters also struggled with their weight. The fad diets that my family cycled through didn't improve my symptoms, and since the concept of whole foods hadn't entered my life yet, I went on the blood pressure medication.

Before long, it became my new normal to be an active high schooler who depended on meds.

Once I went to college, I looked around and realized I was the only one taking blood pressure medication. Something seemed off. I thought, "Geez, I'm in a sea of freshmen and I'm the only one having a hard time riding roller coasters." I would get dizzy when I stood up after lying down! No one else had to bring a blood pressure cuff to college and check their blood pressure on a daily basis. Sometimes, I'd have to head to the nurse's office in between classes. Even with the medication, my readings were still very high. More than once, my blood pressure was 170/110.

I decided there had to be a better way.

So I started to research. I looked into the causes of high blood pressure and educated myself on ways to lower blood pressure—including nutrition. Warning: there is a lot of information out there and not all of it is good.

Over time, I focused on better nutrition in the college cafeteria. I focused on whole foods and exercised simply to remain healthy, instead of training for a competitive event. I felt worlds better and couldn't keep it to myself! I knew I had to help others improve their health as well. My love for athletics and my newfound energy inspired me to become a personal trainer. I started training gym clients one-on-one.

Eventually, I was able to wean myself off the blood pressure medication by changing my lifestyle.

Fast forward a few years. I had married my high school sweetheart, Brandon, who was my best friend since I found him burping the alphabet on the playground in first grade. We became pregnant with our first daughter, Emma, and I successfully stayed fit throughout my pregnancy. Post-delivery, however, I struggled with severe sensitivities. I couldn't figure out what was causing my symptoms! I had stomach pains that left me doubled over in agony while training clients in the gym. It felt like someone was putting knives into my intestines and ripping them apart. In spite of what I thought was "healthy eating" based on my experience as a trainer and previous research, I suspected I had food allergies.

By this time, my stomach pains were negatively impacting not only my career, but my life as a mom, wife, and friend. I found myself canceling gym sessions and missing out on evening activities with friends due to my stomach pains.

They worsened, so back I went to a doctor. I told him I had a major problem and wanted to be tested. He tested me for celiac disease (a disease with an inability to tolerate gluten, which is protein found in wheat, barley, and rye.) And the results came back . . . negative.

Once again, my doctor said, "I don't know what to tell you, Amanda. I'm not really sure what's going on." He sent me home with zero answers and no hope.

Just like the time before, I took matters into my own hands. I started researching the cause of bloating, constipation, digestive issues, and the other symptoms.

Around this time, and shortly before I got pregnant with my son, the paleo lifestyle was gaining popularity. It entailed a gluten-free, dairy-free, and grain-free food log. Colleagues of mine said the lifestyle decreased bloating and Irritable Bowel Syndrome (IBS) symptoms. I decided to try it. Within a matter of days, my symptoms disappeared. I was no longer bloated or having crazy stomach cramps. I was able to do my job as a trainer and web marketing specialist. I felt so much better. Paleo improved my life significantly. The changes were impossible to ignore, so I immediately started implementing a gluten-free, dairy-free, and grain-free lifestyle with my clients.

I maintained paleo through my pregnancy with Cole and postpartum. After delivering baby Cole, I began leading in-person and online bootcamps, in addition to breastfeeding, ramping up my web marketing career, and building a house. I trained clients in person, at home, and online.

It should have been an exciting time. I had a new baby and my career was taking off. However, my health took another turn for the worse. I was living a low-carb lifestyle, I wasn't getting enough fuel or nutrients. In the months after delivering Cole, I was sick. Constantly.

Once again, I went back to the doctor. This time I tested positive for strep throat, and I would go on to test positive a total of five times. My doctor put me on antibiotics for what ended up being a total of sixty one days. I was devastated. Instead of enjoying my baby in the months after his birth, I was hardly able to get through the day, regain my health, and avoid passing my germs to him.

Frustration with my circumstances grew. I was training clients both in the gym and online and was supposed to be the picture of perfect health! At the time, I was even repping popular breakfast shakes that were "all the rage" on social media. A company I had partnered with used intense workouts several times a week, leaving me more tired. When I looked in the mirror, I felt disappointed with the person I saw.

I was tired, depleted, and depressed. Instead of living my best life, I was in survival mode. While preaching to my clients about wellness, promoting mini meals, and protein shakes for breakfast, I struggled with my own health. My clients were hitting plateaus, and I didn't have the answers. I was desperate to improve my own health so I could be a better mom, wife, and trainer. I was just as passionate about empowering my clients to overcome plateaus and develop healthy and sustainable lifestyles.

I knew there had to be a better way, and I knew I could find the solution because I had before. Once again, it was time to take matters into my own hands.

After months of research, I came across the concepts of carb cycling and intermittent fasting (IF) for fat loss. "That's extreme," I said when I first heard about it. In fact, I even told my clients, "Don't try that. It will definitely damage your metabolism."

However, I continued to research the numerous benefits of digestive rest and a shortened feeding window—benefits that include decreased blood glucose levels, increased insulin sensitivity, accelerated fat loss, maintenance of skeletal muscle mass, and an improved immune system. I spoke with a variety of experts on the subject of fasting, read books, listened to podcasts, and read research articles.

I decided to experiment with these strategies in my own life. First with myself on Sundays or while on vacation. Before trying it, I was sure that intermittent fasting would make me feel shaky, hungry, or worse—cause me to pass out. But to my surprise, fasting was easy and I felt amazing. Not only that, my midsection lost a few inches within nine days of implementation.

After personally testing intermittent fasting and carb cycling myself, I saw results. That's when I started to try it with a couple of gym clients who were in plateaus despite consistent workouts and a paleo food log. Much to my excitement, the first client who tried fasting with me lost sixteen pounds in three weeks!

We looked at each other and said, "We're onto something here!"

I experimented with my gym clients further. Instead of simply implementing intermittent fasting with a paleo food log, I added an IIFYM (which is a flexible dieting system that says you can eat whatever you want "If It Fits Your Macros") approach and diligently tracked my macronutrients (macros). I cycled carbohydrates based on the workouts I planned to do each day of the week. The results were astonishing.

After years of straddling the fence between feeling healthy and experiencing near-debilitating health problems, I had cracked the code.

I knew I had to share it.

Why the FASTer Way

In January 2016, I launched the FASTer Way with eleven clients in an online virtual bootcamp. And let me tell you—it was hard to convince those eleven clients to beta test the program. People weren't sure about this extreme-sounding program.

In fact, I had a list of fifty former or current clients that I wanted to get into the program. Everyone was reluctant! I ended up walking around my former workplace and strong-arming several people into trying the FASTer Way. Despite their reluctance, and with big discounts, I signed eleven people into the first testing cycle that incorporated whole food nutrition, intermittent fasting, carb cycling, and a focus on macros, paired with effective workouts.

Although it was a lot of information to consume and a big paradigm shift, my clients absolutely thrived, and I thrived too. Having others doing the program with me took my motivation to a new level and accelerated my own results.

Unfortunately, when I started the FASTer Way, backlash against intermittent fasting was strong. People said it would cause eating disorders, or it wasn't healthy. After all—wellness professionals had been taught and preached for decades that, "Breakfast was the most important meal of the day."

Online haters came out of the woodwork, and many people called me extreme. I was horribly criticized by colleagues, family members, and even friends. Think of the worst thing anyone could say about you, multiply it times ten, and that is the kind of criticism I endured.

But both my clients and I had amazing results and I knew I had to continue growing the program. I knew I'd developed something that solved the problems most popular or expensive programs on the market created, and I couldn't keep it to myself. I said to those first eleven clients, "I need your help to spread the word. I count it an honor and a privilege to work with people you know. So let's go out there and find more people for FASTer Way."

What started with eleven clients is now thousands of clients every month. We quickly scaled the FASTer Way from an idea on a napkin to a multi-million dollar company with tens of thousands of clients and success stories.

In 2017, my vision expanded. Instead of working with clients on my own, I decided to create a certification explaining the science behind the FASTer Way strategies. That way, I could equip and empower other women and men to bring their own clients through the program and earn significant income.

The FASTer Way quickly gained traction and became one of the fastest growing fitness and nutrition programs on the market.

Why? Because it works.

The FASTer Way to Fat Loss is backed by research and science and is empowering tens of thousands of clients all over the world to transform their lives. I've staked my life on it.

There is still a lot of confusion around carbohydrates, fat loss, intermittent fasting, and nutrition. Call it the South Beach diet, Atkins, keto, whatever you want—extreme low-carb lifestyles are literally depleting women of hormones and running them into the ground. At the FASTer Way, we don't eliminate an entire macronutrient, and we don't promote calories in-calories out either.

We promote fat loss for men and women through intermittent fasting, carb cycling, macro tracking, whole food nutrition, and strategic workouts.

Everything I tell you in this book is not only backed by science, but countless success stories. Men and women are transforming their lives with a healthy and sustainable lifestyle. I want you to be successful. I want you to have an incredible transformation, fulfill your purpose, lower your risk of disease, have great energy, and change the world.

Let's dive into that now.

Part One

The FASTer Way Pillars

Chapter One

The WHY Before the HOW

"I've struggled with my weight since I was very young. In 6th grade, I went on my first diet because I had a breakdown in a clothing store fitting room trying on bathing suits with my mom. These struggles only continued, which led to a lot of unhappiness within my own heart. To say my relationship with food was unhealthy is an understatement. That's when the FASTer Way to Fat Loss found me. It's taught me how to fuel my body, how to push my body, and most importantly, how to love my body. I have never felt more confident in how I feel and how I look."

— Brooke L.

In this book, I'm going to share the secret sauce.

The formula that makes the FASTer Way to Fat Loss the best program on the market. However, before we delve into the science, I want to discuss why this matters.

You may be reading this book in a similar spot to where I was several years ago. Exhausted, depleted, frustrated, and desperate for a solution. You may be longing for a healthy, sustainable lifestyle that you can maintain long-term.

The FASTer Way can certainly help—but isn't a magic pill. It's not a quick fix. Yes, with the FASTer Way you will experience accelerated fat loss and results, but it isn't easy. There is a learning curve. In fact, most of my clients feel overwhelmed as they learn the cutting-edge strategies that make the FASTer Way unique and effective. If they hang in there, they receive a sustainable lifestyle that will forever change the way they live.

The frustration of losing and gaining the same amount of weight is proof alone that traditional dieting practices aren't working. It's a helpless feeling when you're doing all the "right" things, but nothing is working.

This Isn't About You

It can be uncomfortable to make a significant lifestyle change. But like I tell my FASTer Way clients, maybe it isn't about *your* comfort. Maybe implementing the FASTer Way lifestyle and becoming healthy once and for all isn't about you.

Perhaps it's about those you will impact.

Your kids, your spouse, your extended family, your church, your co-workers, your community. See, I stepped into the fitness industry and created the FASTer Way for more than to help clients look good in a bikini on the beach. Sure, it's important to empower women and men to be confident, but life is about more than that. When we begin to implement a healthy lifestyle, we have the energy needed to accomplish our goals, fulfill our purpose, and make a massive, positive impact in the world.

Like my good friend Claudia Chan discusses at length in her book, *This is How We Rise*, we must consider how we can *rise to our highest potential and make a positive impact on those around us.*

I believe that starts with good health.

Through the FASTer Way, I equip and empower clients to get well, reduce the risk of disease, and fulfill their purpose with the energy I know they should have.

Now I want to challenge YOU to do the same. A better, more fulfilled life doesn't start and end with wellness. Even in spite of perfect health, you won't ever be fully alive until you find your motivation, your greatest, God-given purpose.

I recommend you read this book and learn the science behind the FASTer Way. I encourage you to implement the FASTer Way in your own life, and I challenge you to rise to your highest potential with the FASTer Way community.

Progress, Not Perfection

Throughout the FASTer Way to Fat Loss, we focus on progress, not perfection. We also celebrate small wins each day and encourage each other to keep pushing forward toward our goals.

Having a positive mindset as you read this book will enable you to overcome doubt and fears. You will routinely hear us say throughout the program and on social media to focus on "progress over perfection." The goal is to experience daily wins (a.k.a. progress) leading to a transformed life.

We believe adopting this mindset will assist you in achieving your goals and, more importantly, see transformation in your life. We continually hear from our clients how the FASTer Way has changed their life.

Just remember, like everyone who attempts change or tries something new, you will have moments that are difficult. I often tell my clients to stop trying to skip the struggle. Challenge is required for change. On average (although this can vary), it takes sixty-six days—or about two months—to form a habit.[1] I have no doubt that if you commit to the FASTer Way lifestyle, you will experience progress, and daily wins leading to a transformed life. Plus, keep in mind, you don't have to make sweeping lifestyle changes all at once to have success. Small steps can add up to giant rewards over time.

YOU'VE GOT THIS,

AND I'M HERE FOR YOU.

Chapter Two

The Secret Sauce:
Behind FASTer Way to Fat Loss

"This way of living changed my life. I found that removing gluten from my diet made me feel better. I found that I love the combination of truly healthy, nutritional foods. I loved tracking my macros to see how it affected my eating choices. I love lifting weights—something that women in my generation were not encouraged to do because it would make us look masculine! How about making us strong? Post-menopausal women need strength so that they can age well, avoid falls, and play with their grandchildren! Through the program, I have been able to lose more than 40 inches from all over my body and drop three pant sizes. And I am still pursuing fitness goals to gain more strength."

—Briane K.

Fat loss isn't really the biggest mystery in the world. Don't let generations of bad information fool you, because we have the answer.

In order to effectively burn fat, we must do the following:
- Eat the right macronutrients, at the right time, for the right reasons.
- Lift heavy to develop lean muscle.
- Engage in fat-burning cardio and high-intensity interval training.
- Maintain the proper mindset.

That is how the FASTer Way is different from other extreme diets or controversial ways of losing weight. The FASTer Way is something you can happily do (without being deprived) for the rest of your life, because of the six components that set us apart.

Intermittent fasting

Carb cycling

Macro tracking

Whole food nutrition

Strategic workouts

Community

In the FASTer Way, you eat the right foods at the right time, do a variety of high intensity interval training (HIIT), lifting, and fat-burning exercises with strategic workouts designed for you, and participate in a community of people ready to help you. All of those requirements to burn fat in the list up there? We hit every one of them.

Let's do a quick review here before we delve into the nitty-gritty behind FASTer Way.

Intermittent Fasting

Before you get too excited or frightened by the word *fasting*, give me a chance to explain it more in-depth. Chapter three is going to go much deeper, but let's do a short review in case it hit your internal panic button.

For our purposes here, let's just be clear: you already fast. Every single day. In fact, your body is always in one of two states: fed or fasted. If you're digesting food, you're in the fed state. That means you have higher levels of insulin in your bloodstream, which makes burning fat a challenge. For 8-12 hours after your body finishes digesting, you're in the fasted state. That means lower insulin and more fat use. That's fasting. Not so scary.

What I like to do with intermittent fasting is to strategically use the boost that the *fasting* state gives us metabolically to burn fat faster.

We'll get into that more later.

Carb Cycling

Carbs have really been through the wringer, haven't they?

Read one article, and you'll hear they're awful and should be eliminated. Read another, and you'll hear they're our preferred source of energy. Carbs cause insulin spikes—and those are good. No, they're bad. Insulin is our friend, then our enemy. Which is right?

And, why am I over here still eating donuts?

Because this is about strategy. Carb cycling is a tool in your belt to help optimize fat loss through increasing thyroid output and controlling hunger. At the FASTer Way, we have high-carb days and low-carb days. If you restrict carbs intensely, over time that adds up to a struggling metabolism. Because, guess what? It's true. Our body does use carbs as brain fuel.[2] But, we need to give it to our body in the right amounts.

Carb cycling ensures fat loss, higher energy levels, and improvement to overall body composition.

Macro Tracking

Macros are the carbohydrates, fat, and protein you're consuming. We don't care about calories around here; we just want the right amount of the right nutrients so we can burn fat. There are a lot of ways to track your macros, from writing it in a journal to plugging it into an app.

Everyone has different goals and different bodies, which also means you should have different macros. In the FASTer Way, you won't have the same macronutrients as other people because we base it on your activity level, your height, your weight, and your health history.

When we decide your macros, this is the only time during the FASTer Way that your weight really matters. Weight loss isn't our goal—fat loss is. When doing exercise, you can increase your muscle mass, which would change your weight, but still lose fat.

MACRONUTRIENT IDEAS

CARBS		PROTEIN		FATS
Apples				Avocado Oil
Bananas	Amaranth	Bison	Chia Seeds	Avocado
Berries	Beans	Chicken	Duck	Butter - non dairy
Brown Rice	Buckwheat	Egg Whites	Eggs	Coconut Milk (full fat)
Carrots	Chickpeas	Fish	Hempseed	
Gluten Free Oats	Lentils	Gluten Free Sausage	Herring	Coconut Butter/ oil
Honey	Millet		Pork	Egg yolk
Pear	Peas	Lean ground beef	Mackerel	Flaxseed
Pumpkin	Quinoa	Protein powder - vegan	Salmon	Nuts
Squash		Scallops	Steak	Nut Butters
Sweet Potatoes		Shrimp	Trout	Olives
Red Potatoes		Turkey		Olive Oil
Veggies				Sesame Oil
				Walnut Oil

Whole Food Nutrition

Whole food nutrition is as simple as it gets. Here's our basic rule: if it comes from the ground or has a mother, it's fair game.

At the FASTer Way, we focus on clean eating. We reduce inflammatory foods like dairy, gluten, and foods that don't make us feel good. Each person requires different foods, so you'll decide which of these foods you'll eat on an individual basis. We're going to be focusing on foods that promote your best health.

Strategic Workouts

Building lean muscle helps us burn fat, so we approach our workouts with the goal to build more lean muscle. We do that through a combination of HIIT, fat-burning cardio, and lifting heavy, as well as an emphasis on rest. Restorative rest!

The FASTer Way to Fat Loss is all about having a healthier body, more energy, better life expectancy, and all the latest science wrapped up in one deliverable package. If you're still with me, that means you're probably ready to learn more.

But it's not enough that I tell you all these incredible stories of other people that have achieved extraordinary things: you need the science. The facts. The studies. If you turn to the back, you'll find a robust references page because science supports the FASTer Way.

You'll see stories of other successful people who have started the FASTer Way throughout this book—with details on all the ways FASTer Way to Fat Loss has changed their lives. Keep reading.

Now it's time to dive deeper.

Community

I could tell you all about these highly effective nutrition strategies, show you the strategic workouts, and send you on your way, but I'd much rather set you up for long-term success.

The key to turning the FASTer Way into a lifestyle and reaching the highest level of success is all in our community.

It has long been known that being in a community can help people change their health behaviors, and now studies show that social support—whether it be in person or online—is crucial for sustainable behavior change[3].

Being a part of a positive community with others who are on the same journey can make you feel less alone and further motivate you to stick with the plan.

TOGETHER, YOU CAN OVERCOME HURDLES, CELEBRATE VICTORIES, AND TRULY GAIN SUPERIOR RESULTS.

Chapter Three

Intermittent Fasting

"Where do I even begin? Before I found FASTer Way to Fat Loss, I was a rundown mom of two toddlers living on fumes. Consumed by daily life and a bad case of emotional eating from said toddlers left me in an unhealthy and unhappy place. My sister introduced me to FASTer Way and convinced me that I could do this. I had great success with Weight Watchers years ago, and she gave me the support and encouragement I needed to sign up for FASTer Way. After starting, I quickly realized that this program was going to be a sustainable lifestyle for me. I lost seventeen pounds and over seventeen inches on my first round. After that, I was hooked! I went on to do five more rounds. I've lost almost sixty pounds. What I've lost is nothing compared to what I've gained. I'm now a happy, healthy wife and mother who is finally thriving in her post-baby body."

—*Susan B.*

The Power of Intermittent Fasting

I'll never forget the day it hit me that I was "onto something" by adding intermittent fasting into my client training programs.

Back in those days, I trained clients at the fitness center located on the campus of my alma mater. Working a full-time day job and training clients in the gym during lunch hours, in the evenings, and on the weekend helped pay the bills. Also . . . I loved the work.

Susan had been a client of mine in the gym for the better part of two years. I had actually started by training her daughters and only began training Susan after she saw the success her daughters experienced.

Susan co-owned a company with her husband and was known for her incredible work ethic, kindness, and generosity. As a small business owner, wife, and mother, she had taken care of everyone else besides herself for far too long. Susan had a significant amount of weight to lose. She was desperate to feel and look her best for the first time in nearly thirty years so she could enjoy her life and have the energy to care for a precious grandbaby on the way.

Susan and I met in the gym two to three times per week and had a blast. I immediately put Susan on a strength training and cardio exercise program and asked her to log her food. Susan saw initial progress after making small changes, but after only a couple months, she hit a plateau.

She and I continued to meet at least two times per week and even trained for a half marathon together when I was pregnant with Cole (which we ran when I was 32.5 weeks pregnant). Even in spite of running a half marathon with me and working extremely hard in the gym, the scale still refused to budge.

The frustration became intense.

The *calories in, calories out* strategies I had been taught and preached for years were not working, and I was determined to find a solution. I came across the concept of intermittent fasting and began to research.

Initially, I thought the concept sounded crazy—even extreme. However, I pulled up some research articles, listened to podcasts, consulted with colleagues who were experts on the subject, and began to personally experiment. To my surprise, I quickly saw positive results and felt amazing.

In fact, after only nine days, my midsection was leaner. I finally burned the stubborn fat around my tummy that held on after delivering baby Cole. I was thrilled!

Naturally, I shared my excitement with Susan in the gym at one of our training sessions, then suggested we try intermittent fasting and a structured meal plan. She agreed, and we started testing it with her.

The first week, we sat together at one of the round tables at the gym and wrote out a simple meal plan focused on whole foods. I added Susan's favorite veggies to her food log, along with grilled chicken, the occasional steak, sweet potatoes, and other simple, whole foods.

Because Susan's job was so demanding and her schedule was packed, we decided to test a sixteen-hour intermittent fasting protocol for most days. (Susan would eat for an eight-hour chunk of the day, then fast for sixteen.) Some days she would start with lunch at the office, but other days she'd break her fast at home with a healthy meal and her family.

To our surprise, fasting was easy for Susan. In fact, it almost became effortless after a few days. We would meet at the gym in the afternoon, and she would report on her progress. Within a week, she came floating into the gym with a smile on her face and a twinkle in her eye. She said, "I feel energized, less bloated, leaner, and in control of my food log for the first time in several months!"

We continued the 16/8 protocol for three weeks, then met at the gym for a leg day workout. Although I have since eliminated weigh-ins, years ago I used to ask clients to hop on the scale every once in a while to track progress.

On this particular day, I asked Susan to step on the scale near the front of the fitness center before our warm-up and pulled up my iPad to check on her weigh-in stats from our last time. She took her shoes off and confidently stepped on the scale. I looked down at the number and could hardly believe my eyes. Susan turned toward me with a huge grin on her face and a giggle.

She had lost sixteen pounds in three weeks!

"I think we're onto something," we exclaimed—practically in unison.

What an incredible feeling to see progress after a plateau. And not just any progress, but significant progress with a seemingly simple strategy. We were overjoyed and couldn't wait to continue the positive momentum.

Turns out, this was just the beginning.

What is Intermittent Fasting?

Although intermittent fasting is a bit of a buzzword in today's health industry, it's truly not something new.

The act of fasting, or abstaining from food for a set time, is an ancient practice used for bringing mental focus and spiritual clarity. However, fasting specifically for physical health is a relatively new concept, and it's spreading fast because the results speak for themselves.

In fact, many religions incorporate fasting, including Judaism, Christianity, and Islam, and have so for thousands of years. Fasting is often seen as a way to control bodily desires and find greater spiritual awakening. Ancient Greeks believed fasting was a medicinal treatment and utilized it when people were sick.

Even one of America's founding fathers, Benjamin Franklin, wrote, "The best of all medicines is resting and fasting." Clearly, fasting has purposes beyond weight loss, which is also why it is such a large component of the FASTer Way program.

If you're intimidated by the F word, I one hundred percent understand and can relate. This is a key strategy, however, that pays big dividends—and it's worth at least trying.

Intermittent fasting encourages the body to burn fat while maintaining lean muscle mass. Because you're mixing periods of higher calorie consumption with lower calorie consumption, you don't get as hungry when you're not eating. And, unlike restricting calories, intermittent fasting doesn't lower the body's basal metabolic rate long-term;[4] in fact, it increases it.[5]

This makes intermittent fasting an incredibly effective weight loss strategy, even for obese people, for two reasons:

1. It has also been shown in scientific studies to be effective even when calories aren't restricted.[6]
2. Intermittent fasting can help people maintain lean muscle mass and lose more fat than normal diets.[7]

After you eat, your body works hard to digest your meal. As the food breaks down in your digestive tract, nutrients are released into your bloodstream—including carbs, protein, and fat. That means your body often has excess fuel.

What happens to it next?

Thanks to insulin, that excess fuel gets stored as fat when it brings glucose into cells to manufacture energy. That energy is used to keep your organs functioning, to support your blood circulating, to maintain your brain at its top game, and to handle any damage caused by toxins and 'wear-and-tear' in your internal systems. During periods of fasting, the body's blood glucose significantly decreases. Once glucose isn't available as fuel, the body will rely on its next preferred fuel source to keep functioning and repairing.

That next-preferred fuel source is fat.

You can literally lose fat while you sleep. When you fast, whether you're awake or asleep, your body has to rely on its energy stores by burning fat and glycogen. Through intermittent fasting, you train your body to burn fat instead of storing it. Intermittent fasting also positively affects the body's hunger hormones: leptin, ghrelin, and insulin. Some studies have shown that intermittent fasting may have an effect on the hypothalamus,[8] which then causes the fat loss benefits we see.

Fad or Fact?

Thanks to recent hype over intermittent fasting, information abounds. Is it another fad? A scientific fact? Or is it a strategy to implement?

I'll tell you this—intermittent fasting is not a fad. It's an eating schedule. (As we discussed, religions have practiced intermittent fasting for both spiritual and health reasons for millennia, so it certainly isn't new.)

We already know that our bodies are in one of two states.

1.   A fasted state, which focuses on repair and healing.[9]
2.   A fed state, which focuses on digesting food.

Of course, we want to repair and heal for longer, which means we need to stay fasted for longer than we're fed. That's where shortening the window frame in which we eat comes into play in a big way.

Let's debunk three hugely false facts from our current culture so you can see the truth about intermittent fasting more clearly.

Breakfast is the most important meal of the day. Debunked. There's actually little trustworthy research to back this claim, which has been heavily propagated by breakfast food companies for years.[10] Research is showing us that skipping breakfast, and eating later in the day allows our body to focus on repair and healing.

Eat six small meals a day. The health and wellness industry has long taught that the best way to keep your metabolism revved up is to eat several small meals. For years, you've probably read that you should eat a big breakfast and snack throughout the day. But, there is actually little to no research to back up this myth.

Fasting will slow my metabolism. Not true . . . *if your calories are not severely restricted within your eating window.* As long as you eat enough within the allotted window of time (which is anywhere from 6-8 hours a day), you'll see no issues with your metabolism slowing down.

Let's talk more about your metabolism and intermittent fasting.

Intermittent Fasting and Metabolism

Metabolism has little to do with eating periods. It's most closely related to muscle mass. The more lean muscle you have, the faster your metabolism will be. This is why we utilize strength training workouts in the FASTer Way, so we can effectively build muscle that will increase our metabolic rate.

The American Journal of Clinical Nutrition[11] published a study in 2000 where subjects went through four days of fasting to determine the impact on resting energy expenditure. (Resting energy expenditure is simply the amount of energy your body needs to carry out its most basic functions.)

This study found that a person's resting energy expenditure, or their metabolism, *increased for the first three days*. In a similar study, subjects utilized an alternate day fasting protocol for twenty-two days. That study found that subjects saw *no decrease in their resting metabolic rate*[12].

There are countless other studies that provide the same kind of results: fasting has no negative effect on metabolic rate, but has significant positive effects on overall health and wellness.

As we allow our body the time it needs to rest and repair itself, while building lean, calorie-burning muscle through effective workouts, we see an increased metabolic rate and a significant change to our overall body composition.

Intermittent Fasting Protocols

Before you jump into this without question, let's review the different hour splits you can use with intermittent fasting, as well as the reasoning behind them. There are some I absolutely recommend—and others I don't.

Like everything in the FASTer Way to Fat Loss, your plan should reflect your needs and your goals. Here are a few approaches to intermittent fasting:

1. **12/12.** This is a perfect place to start—at twelve hours of fasting and feeding. With this schedule, you can begin at and continue with a fairly normal schedule because almost all your fast will happen at night, and this still allows an early morning, traditional breakfast.

2. **16/8.** This is where you fast for sixteen hours and then feed for eight hours. This may look like you eating breakfast at 10:00 am, then dinner at 6:00 pm with your family, and nothing from the

time you finish dinner to the time you start breakfast. Alternately, you may prefer to break your fast at 8:00 am with breakfast, and eat dinner before 4:00 pm. This is a very common split and what we implement in the FASTer Way program. I find this the easiest, most sustainable approach that still gives results. Luckily, most fasting occurs when you're sleeping!

3. **20/4.** This is when you fast for twenty hours. I like the 20/4 split particularly when I'm on vacation or know I'm going to have a big meal later in the day. This allows me to eat less food earlier, then enjoy more of that food later without giving my body too much.

4. **Multi-day fasts. (3, 14, 21 days, etc.)** There are certain reasons and circumstances to do these, but we don't use these as part of our methodology. Of course, if you're thinking of doing something this extensive, always speak with your doctor or a trained professional. Extensive fasts can do greater damage if your body is already in a place that isn't ready for it.

The 24-Hour Fast

Many people do a 24-hour fast every other day, or they do 24-hour fasts every week, typically on the weekend.

A lot of research has been done here, particularly for women, that may show that frequent fasting for that long may have a negative hormonal effect. Frequent 24-hour fasts are not suggested for women, especially every other day fasts.

The FASTer Way methodology does incorporate the occasional 24-hour fast because it allows your body to be at complete digestive rest. When the body isn't focused on digesting food, delivering/storing nutrients, or burning it for fuel, it can then focus on other important bodily processes like cellular repair.

Apoptosis (normal cell death) and autophagy (the destruction of damaged or redundant cellular components) are critical for healthy regeneration. This is why fasting is so powerful when it comes to reducing the risk of cancer[13] and Alzheimer's.[14] The damaged cells that contribute to disease are being removed from the body in a totally natural way.

This also allows the body to burn any extra glycogen and then dip into its fat stores for its main fuel throughout the day. Fasting also helps with lipid (fat) metabolism, stabilizes blood sugar levels, keeps insulin levels consistent, improves gut health,[15] and improves body composition.

Whatever protocol you implement, we do not recommend you try this on your own because of the potential negative effect on hormone health. (Some women end up significantly limiting their calories without meaning to, and that can cause more problems.) Join the FASTer Way lifestyle so you can learn the right, safest approach.

The Scientific Benefits Behind Intermittent Fasting

It's one thing for me to tell you that this works, but, more importantly, science backs me up. Studies show that intermittent fasting appears to work because of two mechanisms: reduced oxidative damage and increased cellular stress resistance. Intermittent fasting helps your body deal with stress. Fasting triggers the process of autophagy, which breaks down and recycles dysfunctional proteins and cellular debris. Specifically, here's what intermittent fasting can do for you:

1. **Fat loss.** This is the obvious number one benefit that everyone is talking about. Everybody is excited about fat loss—and for good reason. Intermittent fasting is shown to help increase fat loss, even for obese people,[16] and is shown to be just as—or possibly more effective—than calorie restriction alone.[17] Numerous benefits piggyback off having less fat in your body, which enables a naturally healthier system.[18]

2. **Natural detoxing.** It's important to drink a lot of water if you're fasting because our body is detoxing. Water gives it the opportunity to continue to flush out all the toxins that we acquire, whether it's through food, pollution, water, or other means. I use my mornings (I'm on a 16/8 split) to drink a lot of tea and a lot of water (at room temp so it's readily available for my body to use) to optimize my fast.

3. **Cellular repair.** Intermittent fasting activates pathways in our cells so that they handle stress better—right down to DNA repair at the mitochondrial level[19]. It also helps our brain get rid of the dead cells that aren't needed[20].

4. **Decreases insulin.** Not only is this the best news for people with diabetes—whether you're type 1 or type 2—but for anyone engaged in wanting to lose weight. Lower insulin allows even greater fat loss. We simply can't lose weight when we have high insulin levels because insulin is also known as the *fat storage hormone.*

5. **Increased insulin sensitivity.** Another hormonal perk from fasting! This is especially important for women with polycystic ovarian syndrome (PCOS) as well as type 2 diabetes.

6. **Lowers risk of diabetes and Alzheimers.** Intermittent fasting is becoming part of the widespread treatment for type 2 diabetes because it not only lowers insulin levels and increases sensitivity,[21] but it can decrease the risk of type 2 diabetes even forming in those susceptible. Intermittent fasting can help lower your risk for Alzheimer's[22] as well because fasting is shown to prevent or address the disease process. It's been made clear lately that being in a fed state negatively affects the brain, specifically later in life.

7. **Reduces inflammation.** Remember how intermittent fasting activates our cells to handle stress better? That directly influences inflammation in our body.[23] Our better functioning cells now handle oxidative stress much better, which means our inflammation drops.

8. **Improves hormone profile.** In addition to reducing insulin levels, intermittent fasting has been shown to raise the amount of human growth hormone[24] in the body. Higher levels of this hormone are linked with improved fat burning and muscle gain, among other benefits.

9. **Increases life expectancy.** Intermittent fasting doesn't only add life to your years, but it appears to add years to your life, too. Studies show that intermittent fasting diets may lengthen your lifespan.[25]

10. **Maintenance of skeletal muscle mass.** Intermittent fasting helps with the maintenance of muscle, especially when combined with the strength training implemented in FASTer Way.[26] In other words, some people are worried that fasting causes us to go into starvation mode and wear down our muscles for energy. When done right, it doesn't cause our muscles to break down.

11. **Reduces risk of coronary disease.** Studies show that intermittent fasting can improve certain health markers linked with a reduced risk of heart disease. Intermittent fasting can also help lower body weight, accelerate fat loss, especially around the midsection, and reduce total and low-density lipoprotein cholesterol (LDL or "bad" cholesterol) levels, all of which can slash heart disease risk.[27]

Integrating Intermittent Fasting

Fasting doesn't have to be complicated.

If you're in good health, and you've gotten the go-ahead from your doctor, you can try the 16/8 protocol (though I highly suggest doing it as part of the FASTer Way program rather than on your own). This allows for your body to daily reset itself, without feeling too restrictive, which makes it a strategy that is easy to sustain long-term. There are times when I have clients do a 24-hour fast to give the body a more significant rest period, but for the most part, we stick to the 16/8 protocol.

When you start, do the 16/8 on a Sunday or on vacation. No, I'm not kidding! You can fast on vacation. Start your fasted window immediately after dinner the night before, then skip breakfast, and give yourself the luxury of a big, delicious meal later without overstuffing yourself.

Once you've tried intermittent fasting on a weekend, try it again on Monday. If waiting until lunch is too much, that's fine. Start eating at 10:00 am, then keep moving it back until you've reached a sixteen-hour fasting window.

Note: it's important to start it immediately after dinner the night before, so you've already completed about 12-13 hours of the fast while you're sleeping. Also, the word breakfast literally means break the fast. Your break the fast meal is important. We want to be sure that when you do break your fast, we're consuming carbs, fats, and proteins to give your body the nutrients that it needs. I break my fast around noon, then maintain a eight-hour feeding window so I can eat dinner with my family in the evening.

Thriving Through Your Fast

Here are a few tips to make sure you're optimizing your time while fasting and really thriving through it. If we take advantage of what our body is doing, we can make amazing things happen.

Besides, breaking my fast around noon takes pressure off in the morning. It allows me to get my kiddos and myself ready without all the stress of preparing my meal, because all I have to do is drink some water and stay hydrated.

1. During your fasting window, consume water, herbal tea, black coffee, etc. Nothing with creamer or dairy additives.
2. Track your macros. We are not restricting calories, so it's important to get in all of your macronutrients (proteins, fats, and

carbohydrates) during your eating window. Through the FASTer Way, we teach our clients how to calculate and track macronutrients which is a key component of their success. The focus should be on whole foods, not processed options.

3. Work out while fasted, if possible. This will maximize your hormonal output and increase your metabolic rate. However, if you can't get your workout in during that window, don't stress.
4. Have a plan for what you'll eat during your eating window. Stay busy while fasting. Being prepared is the best way to ensure your success!
5. Eat enough the night before, but make sure you only eat until you're 80% satisfied. You shouldn't be overfull. Be satiated, not stuffed. You will eat again! A fast is no reason to overstuff yourself.
6. Drink a ton of water through the morning. This is important to help the detoxing process along. The same signal that tells us we're hungry also tells us we're dehydrated. We're often simply dehydrated instead of hungry.
7. Eat enough of the right food in between fasts. If you maintain a calorie deficit, or are not consuming enough macros, you'll create more issues. There's a right supply of food in order to thrive and fuel through the day. You must be sure that you're eating enough.
8. Replace your traditional morning breakfast with a different activity. Instead of eliminating it, replace that time with something else, like a workout, meditation, or a pedicure. Who doesn't love an occasional pedicure?
9. Branched-chain amino acids (BCAAs), which are three of your essential amino acids that act as building blocks for your muscles, can help preserve your energy, and some participants in FASTer Way swear by them.

Now test your fasting process through the week, and be sure to listen to your body. Do you need more or less? How are you feeling? Not drinking enough water and not eating enough during your eating window are two of the biggest mistakes. To get the full benefits, you must properly hydrate and fuel your body.

I know this sounds difficult, but I promise it gets easier as you try, and the members of our FASTer Way community can attest to this. You can do hard things! Prove to yourself that you can do it, and that it's actually easier than you thought.

Surround Yourself with a Community

Although this isn't a deal-breaker right away, it will be eventually. I want you to be aware of my last piece of advice when it comes to fasting:

Don't go it alone.

Here's why.

The 16/8 protocol without any other intention can be detrimental. You may do great at fasting, but be sabotaging yourself in other ways. Maybe you have adrenal fatigue (no, you shouldn't be doing a lot of fasting with that!), and you don't realize it. Maybe your thyroid is tired and you need to make some other changes first. If you add fasting onto an already overtaxed system, you're asking for trouble. Then you're going to try fasting, think it's a hoax because it doesn't work, and lose out on all the amazing benefits. Some people try intermittent fasting on their own, but don't consume enough food in their feeding window — or they don't consume the right macronutrient ratios — and end up not having success.

That's why the FASTer Way is so special.

We create the community and the expertise that people need to be successful with these strategies. You are never alone, and there's nothing you'll ever have to figure out on your own.

Intermittent fasting has truly changed my life for the better. I have never felt stronger, leaner, or more energetic, and I want this for you too.

Special Considerations

1. Do NOT dive in, particularly if you're being treated for full-blown adrenal fatigue or hypothyroidism. In those cases, you need to start with the 12/12 protocol and gradually work toward longer fasts. Ask your doctor, and have them advise you. Your naturopathic doctor may also have an opinion on when you break your fast through the day, so be sure to weigh in on what they say first. The last thing we want to do is create more damage.
2. If you have type 2 diabetes, I would advise you to try the 12/12 and work up to the 16/8. Of course, it goes without saying—always consult with your doctor first.
3. If you're on medication that you have to take 12 hours apart *with food*, then modify your fast to fit your doctor's requirements. (Not the other way around.)

Frequently Asked Questions

Is intermittent fasting okay for everyone?

Yes, intermittent fasting is okay for everyone, but I always recommend a visit with your doctor before you start. We don't recommend it for children, but people of all races, genders, ages, and backgrounds can safely practice intermittent fasting.

What can be consumed during the fasting period?

Anything under fifty calories, that contains no fiber, and is preferably unsweetened, will not trigger the digestion process. Avoid sugar, honey, maple syrup, and most artificial sweeteners[28], as they will elicit an insulin response, which halts fat-burning and the production of growth hormone. Most people can use a small amount of Stevia, but I advise clients to use liquid Stevia extract or uncut Stevia powder (most Stevia powders are mixed with other ingredients). The last hours of the fast are a great time to drink a lot of water.

What if this is too hard for me?

Many people find this portion of the program challenging. If you're having a hard time, begin with a smaller window, and increase the window as your comfort level increases. For example, do 3-4 days of a 12-hour fast, then bump that to a 14-hour fast, and then finally a 16-hour fast. The goal is a long-term lifestyle change, so easing into this is incredibly wise.

Can I still take supplements when intermittent fasting?

Yes, you can. But it's also beneficial to give your body an occasional break from supplements to reduce the chance for sensitivities.

Why am I always cold while fasting?

Fasting increases adipose tissue blood flow (blood flow to your body fat). Because of this, your blood rushes away from fingers and toes into fat stores, leaving your hands and feet feeling a bit colder than normal.

Frequently Asked Questions

Are headaches normal while fasting?

For some people, yes, but not for everyone. Headaches can occur during fasted periods and are often confused with dehydration headaches. While drinking more water will not hurt you, dehydration is not typically the cause of headaches during fasting. Instead, it's more likely that your body is feeling "withdrawal-like" symptoms similar to those you might feel when giving up caffeine or sugar. Headaches should not last beyond your first few fasts, and can be treated the same way you would treat them while not in a fasted state.

Does intermittent fasting negatively impact female hormones or fertility?

Preliminary studies[29] in rats show intermittent fasting to have a negative impact on fertility rates. However, those studies all use an alternate day fasting protocol and no comparable studies in humans have been conducted at this time. With an alternate day protocol, the likelihood of someone under eating is significant. This type of restrictive caloric intake will undoubtedly have a negative impact on female hormone levels. That's why at FASTer Way we don't practice calorie restriction. Instead, we aim to take in a healthy number of calories during the feeding window.

I have hypothyroidism or adrenal fatigue. Can I do intermittent fasting?

Yes, but ease into intermittent fasting with a 12/12 protocol, and practice the 16/8 protocol as able. Stick to the list of approved foods, eliminate gluten and dairy, and consume enough complex carbohydrates. Be especially mindful of the balance between stress and rest, focus on sleep, and get adequate sunlight within two hours of the sun rising.

I work night shifts. Can I still fast?

Of course, but because of that, we have to switch things up. One of my good friends works night shift and manages it on a day-by-day basis. Most of you will prefer to break your fast around noon, which is great.

Chapter Four

Whole Food Nutrition

"Before FASTer Way, I had completely lost the ability to feel like myself. I put on quite a bit of weight, had gut health issues, and really didn't like myself. I was completely confused about which foods were healthy and which were not. I had become afraid of food and never enjoyed anything. A few weeks into my first round with Faster Way, I knew this was the thing that would help me. My bloating went away, gut health issues resolved, and the inflammation disappeared. I started feeling like me again."

—Stacie M.

Despite the ease of accessing information these days and the development of new research in food science, I continue to hear incorrect advice, even from doctors, about nutrition. Myths abound in popular culture and mainstream media that will lead you down false paths. So many people have opinions and ideas that it's easy to get pulled in every direction and question your own judgment.

That's how FASTer Way is different.

We didn't pull one set of data and create an entire paradigm on it. We watched, tested, and tried out cutting edge advances in the field of nutrition and brought them into a program. Plus, you don't have to rely on me. You can take the data from the tens of thousands of clients we've worked with to see what their experience is.

But really . . . this program starts with changing the way you eat. Our focus through the FASTer Way to Fat Loss is nutrition. Of course, our workouts will help you accelerate and maximize your results, but many of my clients simply follow the nutrition cycle and lose weight through the food they eat.

The *real* food they eat.

What Is Whole Food Nutrition?

The FASTer Way to Fat Loss is a whole food-based program because whole foods are the best way to eat and nourish the body.

Whole food nutrition is self-explanatory—when we're eating whole foods, we're eating real food. None of this frankenfood you get with eating fast food all the time. (Marshmallow fluff, anyone?) No preservatives, additives, or fake sugars. It may sound scary, but it doesn't have to be. I promise, this is a sustainable way to live.

The bulk of your nutrition should consist of foods found in their most natural state. Whole foods have few ingredients, are easily pronounced, have not been modified, and are not processed. They have no added sugars or chemicals.

They are simply . . . whole.

Of course, you could eat all processed food and still hit your macro goals, but it won't be nearly as healthy as a whole food diet because you'd be missing out on very important micronutrients. Whole foods generally have more micronutrients than processed foods. While you may not be worried about or impressed by micronutrients, make no mistake about it—these micronutrients include vitamins, minerals, antioxidants, and other bioactive compounds that are good for our bodies.

Really good for our bodies.

Whole foods are also generally higher in fiber. Both soluble (that means it develops a gel-like consistency with water) and insoluble (doesn't react with water) fiber are incredibly important for your health. Soluble fiber helps keep you healthy by reducing cholesterol, and insoluble fiber decreases constipation. Both fibers may also help you lower your blood pressure and reduce inflammation.

Whole foods include but are not limited to:

Fruits	Herbs and spices	Beans
Vegetables	Nuts	Legumes
Meats		

Why Whole Food Nutrition?

For over a decade, I struggled with PCOS.

It caused irregular menstrual cycles and a whole host of other unpleasant issues. When my husband Brandon and I decided to expand our family, my doctor said, "It's going to be difficult to conceive, Amanda. I'm sorry."

My heart ached. We wanted a family, but I didn't want to go this route. To help us have a child, my doctor put me on a series of medications once again. With Clomid, among other things, I struggled through the regimen, the hormonal swings, and the inherent difficulty of getting pregnant with PCOS. Eventually, I was able to conceive my oldest daughter Emma and later my son, Cole. Both of them required Clomid and fertility assistance.

After creating and living the FASTer Way and committing to whole food nutrition, tracking macros, intermittent fasting, carb cycling, and more, my cycles regulated. My hormones balanced out. I felt better than I ever had before.

Without medications!

About fifteen months after living the FASTer Way lifestyle, I noticed that I started to feel bloated. *Do I need to adjust my macros?* I thought. I often tell my clients to ask themselves a series of questions prior to adjusting macros, so I dove in.

1. Have my measurements changed and/or are my clothes fitting different? *Still looking lean and fitting into my clothes . . . but definitely feeling bloated. My pants are getting slightly tighter around the midsection. Hmm.*
2. Have I been getting consistent, good quality sleep? *Yep.*
3. Am I stressed, feeling overtrained, or neglecting to care for myself? *At this time—nope!*

4. Am I approaching my period? *Yes . . . but with the FASTer Way, I rarely have PMS symptoms.*

5. Am I properly hydrated, and/or have I been indulging in food that is higher in sugar, salt, or alcohol? *Yes, I'm hydrated, and I've been sticking with the FASTer Way list of approved foods and keeping it clean.*

The conclusion seemed clear: my hormones must be out of balance.

I scheduled an appointment with a functional medicine doctor who recommended comprehensive hormonal blood work. A few days later I had my blood drawn—it cost me $650—and I remember hoping she would quickly find the answer.

Turns out I could have saved myself both time and money by taking an at-home-pregnancy-test.

To my surprise, I was pregnant!

My pregnancy happened naturally with Lily, which became the best surprise of my life thus far. Since then, we have affectionately called this program the FASTer Way to Fertility!

Thankfully, I enjoyed a healthy pregnancy and continued the FASTer Way all the way to the end—with a safe delivery. The first month postpartum was the best month of my life! Thousands of new clients were starting the FASTer Way, so I immediately re-committed to the FASTer Way list of approved foods with a focus on whole food nutrition the following Monday. I consumed nuts, fruits, lean meat, lots of veggies, and more.

The whole foods gave me the fuel needed to breastfeed and maintain a wonderful supply. Of course, the first four weeks of Lily's life came with some challenges, but I loved feeling confident in my nutrition plan and choices. Having that solid ground beneath me at a challenging time for our family was wonderful.

After that, I consumed whole foods as if her life depended on it. And you know what—it did. Still does! I meticulously planned out my food log and considered my food choices. I chose nutrient-dense whole foods high in good carbs, good fats, and lean protein. Thanks to that, I had a wonderful supply of breast milk.

Whole food nutrition not only helped my recovery from one of the most draining, dangerous stages of a woman's life, but also served my daughter and my family. Thanks to whole food nutrition, my family enjoys greater health and success.

The more intentional I am about whole food nutrition, and living the

FASTer Way lifestyle, the better. Not only for me, but for my family. To find my motivation to remain committed to eating the right foods, I don't have to look any further than my kiddos. As part of the whole food nutrition, the FASTer Way lifestyle advocates for also getting rid of anything that doesn't serve us—like gluten, dairy, and alcohol. Let's go a little deeper into why.

Gluten

Gluten is a protein found in wheat, spelt, rye, and barley. You'll find gluten in most baked goods (unless they're specifically marked as gluten-free) because gluten gives breads and other similar foods their spongy or gooey consistency.

During the FASTer Way to Fat Loss program, I encourage clients to eat mostly gluten-free because of the way gluten products are genetically modified, which often leads to inflammation, stomach discomfort, aches and pains, breakouts, and fatigue.

While the FASTer Way to Fat Loss is based on a carb cycling philosophy, we are very specific about the types of carbs we consume. Those found in fruits and veggies are significantly better for the digestive system than those found in processed carbs like bread and grains.

Whole foods are often naturally gluten-free, especially the healthiest whole foods, veggies and fruits.

Dairy

Let's get one thing straight: cow's milk is for baby cows.

Cows produce milk for the same reason humans do—to feed their young. The nutrients in a cow's milk are the perfect nutrition for a calf, just as a human mother's milk is perfect nutrition for her child. However, humans do not have the same nutritional needs as calves. The exact balance of a cow's milk is not the same as a human's.

Also—milk contains a lot more than milk.

A significant amount of antibiotics is given to cows to prevent them from getting infections. Those antibiotics filter into a cow's milk supply, tainting what we find in our cups and cereal bowls. Antibiotics given to farm animals are also a major contributor to the rise of antibiotic-resistant bacteria, which can have major impacts on human health.

In addition, cows in the U.S. are pumped full of growth hormones, which, when consumed by humans, raise our IGF-1 levels. Increased IGF-1 levels have been linked to prostate, colon, and breast cancers.[30] When you pour yourself a glass of milk, you are pouring a little bit of milk, and a significant amount of hormones and antibiotics.

Some milk products are labeled in a way that confuses clients. If products are labeled "lactose-free," "dairy-free," "contains milk proteins," or "whey based," then they should still be considered dairy products. Products that contain parts of milk, such as whey or proteins, still contain dairy. Milk that has had lactose (sugar) removed is still considered dairy.

In an article about going dairy-free, Alisa Fleming cites a well-known study saying, "According to the landmark Harvard study of approximately 78,000 female nurses, women who consumed greater amounts of calcium from dairy foods had a significantly increased risk of hip fractures, while no increase in fracture risk was observed for the same levels of calcium intake from non-dairy sources[31]."

This wasn't the only study to stumble upon these findings. Several other studies conducted over the years have shown countries with the highest rates of osteoporosis are also the highest consumers of dairy products.

Many women ask if the issue with dairy is truly with dairy products, or with the manipulation of those products in today's market. It's the manipulation. This leaves the door open for both organic or raw milk as alternatives to the modified milk we find in grocery stores. However, in the FASTer Way, we truly believe cow's milk is meant to be consumed by calves, not humans. Most of us stop producing lactase—the enzyme responsible for breaking down lactose—by the age of five. Our bodies aren't meant to consume milk much longer than when we are weaned.

With so many great-tasting, viable, healthy dairy replacement options on the market, I highly recommend that clients try to live as dairy-free as possible. And, while this isn't true across the board, it is true that for many people, milk causes significant digestive issues.

According to Dr. Mark Hyman,[32] "About 75 percent of the world's population is genetically unable to properly digest milk and other dairy products—a problem called lactose intolerance."

The majority of FASTer Way participants report feeling less bloated and experience fewer digestive problems after cutting out dairy.

Trust me; it's worth it.

Alcohol

If you want maximum results, avoid it. Alcohol can actually stop your body from burning fat properly, negating all of the hard work you're doing at the gym and in the kitchen.

Alcohol is the first fuel to burn in your body[33] (even before carbohydrates), so fat burning comes to a halt when alcohol is consumed. It contains no nutrients, and at seven calories per gram, it supplies almost twice as many calories as protein and carbs, and only two fewer than fat. Keep in mind that many alcoholic beverages also contain calories from other sources (like mixed drinks).

Alcohol tends to have appetite-stimulating effects, which means you need to be mindful of food when you drink. If you absolutely *must* have a drink, stick to just one! If you choose to have a drink, aim to have it as your treat on leg day. Stay away from sugar.

Integrating Whole Food Nutrition

It's one thing to appreciate the benefits of whole food nutrition, but a whole other game entirely to integrate it into your life. Here are a few ground rules to keep it simple when it comes to starting out with whole foods.

If it came from the ground or has a mother, it's fair game.
Get rid of the gluten.
Get rid of the dairy.
Focus on veggies and fruits.

I believe in bio-individuality. We're all different, and our bodies need different things. There is no cookie cutter approach to health. The FASTer Way provides a fantastic kickstart with highly effective guidelines, and sometimes we have to make adjustments. Do what serves your body the best.

For example, I can't eat a lot of almonds or much broccoli because my body doesn't process it correctly. Maybe you can't handle Brussels sprouts. As you move through this program, you'll gain a better understanding of what helps fuel your day, and you'll have more information. I urge you to pay careful attention to your symptoms, noting if they occur after eating certain foods. Your certified coach will guide you through this process so you can find the foods that not only fuel you well, but also help you to feel your best.

Keep in mind—you don't have to suffer or be miserable in order to lose weight. You don't have to do "insane workouts" and undereat or be hangry.

Before we close this out, let's debunk two myths that circle around the fitness world. If you give into these, they will stall your success!

Myth #1: CICO (Calories In, Calories Out)

So many people still preach the calorie-counting philosophy of eat less, exercise more, and you'll lose weight. Even most doctors these days continue to believe in the theory that weight loss is as simple as consuming fewer calories than you burn.

It's not.

With all the intricate hormonal processes that go behind losing weight (and gaining greater health), I see exactly what's happening. We follow their advice to "count calories, and eat less than you burn," but still find ourselves depleted and frustrated. Then we hit a plateau and crash mid-afternoon from lacking energy.

I want to prevent that!

We stop these problems through whole food nutrition. FASTer Way ensures you don't restrict your calories or obsessively worry over them because it just doesn't work.

But you probably already know that.

Myth #2: Eat Less in a Plateau

If you want to burn fat, lose weight, and establish a long-term lifestyle, eat more of the right foods.

Here's the deal: CICO will work temporarily if you had been over-consuming on macros and under-exercising. If you were used to eating 2,300-3,000 calories per day without exercise, bringing the macros down and moving more can yield short-term results.

But most of you have probably been trying to eat healthy for a long time. You've watched your portions and worked out until your bones ached, but the weight isn't coming off. It seems impossible to get significant results. This means that you're in the dreaded plateau.

This isn't time for restricting your food intake.

You need to eat more.

Eat more fruits, veggies, fats, and proteins in order to see results long-term. In my program, when we hit a plateau, we bump up the macros. Guess what? Weight loss follows. Of course, some clients don't listen to me. They don't increase macros, and they also stay in the plateau. Then they go on vacation, eat more, enjoy themselves, and come home to find they've lost weight.

A plateau often means you're not supporting your body or balancing your hormones. If you really use common sense, you'll be able to see that a long-term calorie deficit, maintaining stress, and working out a lot means that something is going to break.

That something is your thyroid.

Many times, we're not eating enough to support thyroid, hormones, and stress levels. That's the problem! It's not that you're overeating. You're not consuming enough to support your body. You're actually under-consuming the nutrients that your body needs.

You'll hear from doctors, industry professionals, and other trends to eat less. That can be a temporary answer, but it isn't a long-term solution.

There's a place for deficit dieting, but not nearly as much as it has been touted up until now.

Whole foods will significantly improve your energy levels, reduce your stomach discomfort, and help you feel considerably better overall. However, participating in a gluten-free, dairy-free lifestyle is not a deal-breaker for the program. You can still fit gluten and dairy into your macros; just try to do so sparingly.

Frequently Asked Questions

Can vegans participate in FASTer Way?

It's definitely possible to participate in the FASTer Way to Fat Loss if you're vegan! In fact, because we suggest avoiding dairy, vegans are a step ahead in some ways. Follow the same macros and calorie goals as non-vegans, and plan ahead carefully for low-carb day, since many vegans tend to have high-carb diets. Vegan protein shakes, peanut and other nut butters, tofu, and tempeh are all great protein options that vegans could use to meet their macros. We also have a wonderful FASTer Way Vegan Cookbook.

Will I gain weight eating all this food?

You will not gain weight on my program. I often hear people say, "I'm eating more than I ever have. I'm going to gain weight on this program." Four weeks later, they are feeling great and getting leaner.

Can I move my feeding window?

Absolutely. Some of you might prefer to do your feeding window a little earlier in the day. You may want to break your fast at 7:00 AM, per usual, and then eat for eight hours.

Can I still have wine?

We limit alcohol intake, but you can still have it in moderation through the FASTer Way.

Chapter Five

Nutrients and IIFYM

Nutrients—Macros and Micros

Our nutrient profiles break into two aspects: macronutrients and micronutrients.

The three main macro (large) nutrients that comprise our diet are carbs, fat, and protein. They typically take up the bulk of what you eat. This is yet another spot where the FASTer Way differs from other programs, because we don't cut out an entire macronutrient. (Like going zero-carb or low-fat).

The body requires complex regulation. If you have too much fat, we don't function optimally. If you don't have enough carbohydrates, you're going to run yourself out of hormones. If you don't have enough protein, you're not going to be able to develop lean calorie-burning muscle, which will, in turn, improve or increase your metabolism. We need to be sure that we're having enough, but not too much.

At FASTer Way, we're going to help you find and adjust to the right macronutrient profile for your body.

Let's review each macronutrient; then we'll talk more about micronutrients.

Carbs

Our body was made to use carbohydrates for energy and fuel. Carbohydrates are important because they are the body's primary (and preferred) fuel source. Most people need to consume approximately 45-50% carbs. Unfortunately, our modern fast-food culture has led us far astray from the types—and amounts—of carbs that are good for us.

Not all carbs are created equal.

With whole food nutrition, we focus on complex carbohydrates such as beans, peas, sweet potatoes, oats, and rice. Complex carbs are digested more slowly than simple carbs (which means they provide longer-lasting satiety) and should be the main focus of carbohydrate intake. Limit simple carbohydrates such as honey and pure maple syrup, and avoid refined sugar. Enjoy any fruit desired, as long as it fits into the carb cycle/macro count for any given day.

Avoid refined carbohydrates, especially gluten-containing varieties.

A Note on Keto

There's no doubt that the ketogenic diet (also known as keto) is a hot topic right now. It's very trendy—and for good reason. The primary emphasis of the keto diet is eating a very low percentage of carbohydrates in your diet in order to encourage your body to burn fat instead of sugar. It has high fat, moderate protein, low carbs, usually with a 70/25/5 (fats/protein/carb) ratio. The emphasis here is also on healthy fats that fuel brain and body, such as avocado and coconut oils.

There certainly are undeniable benefits to this method of eating, which we won't go into here with great detail. Keto does reduce the risk of type 2 diabetes, cancer, and heart disease, as well as neurological disorders.

I believe the keto diet is best suited for people who have a significant amount of weight to lose and are very sedentary. It can help you lose weight fast so you can move more easily.

But . . . that's not quite how we work at FASTer Way. Over here, we like to leverage keto strategies while still consuming carbs. If you're coming from the keto camp, don't worry. You can ease into carbs if you don't want to do it all at once. In fact, we are the perfect transition plan if you're coming from keto, because we have low-carb days.

One of my coaches had her mother go through the program and had this to say about the experience.

> *"My mom has considerable weight to lose (70-80lbs). For the past twenty years, she has been sedentary and low energy and addicted to sugar, eating powdered donuts for breakfast every day. In addition to being addicted to sugar, she has also been undereating. After two small strokes, she decided to try the keto diet.*
>
> *After two months on keto, she was already looking for an alternative. She felt very deprived and didn't enjoy eating heavy, fatty foods all day every day, so she still found herself undereating. She decided to join the FASTer Way to Fat Loss after I became certified, and she was looking forward to carb cycling so she could still eat her favorite keto foods a few days a week. but not have to eat them every day.*
>
> *Although she struggled to adjust at first, she overcame her sugar cravings and no longer craves the powdered donuts in the morning. She tried Pilates after being sedentary for twenty years, her cholesterol dropped forty points, and she lost twenty-five pounds! Her bloodwork is the best it's ever been.*

*She wasn't perfect, and it took her weeks to build up to her
recommended calories, and yet she is a true success story.
A little bit of progress each week is paying off for her in big
ways.*

People who come to my program from keto can't get over their
energy level because you need some carbs. We are the solution for those
who feel low-carb options aren't for them.

Fats

Now is not the time to be scared of the word *fat*.

Once upon a time, we went through a time of terror about fats.
Thanks to faulty information, we believed that fat was the enemy. After
that, fat-free and low-fat alternatives to almost everything flooded the
markets, which is part of the reason we have the massive obesity spike
now. When you pull fat from a food, you add lots of sugar and create an
even bigger processed issue.

With whole food nutrition in the FASTer Way, we aren't afraid of fats—
just as we aren't solely focused on them either. We emphasize good fats.
Coconut oil. Avocado oil. (Both have properties that protect your heart.[34])
Get rid of the highly processed fats like soybean (aka vegetable oil) and
peanut oil because they increase inflammation in your body and aren't
good for you.

Fat is a fantastic form of fuel, a protective mechanism that our body
employs, as well as a storage facility for vitamins and minerals. In fact, fat
is essential for our brains.

Protein

Protein is used to build and repair tissues, and it's even a source of
energy for the body, though not an ideal one. The body will literally start
consuming its own muscle, which we don't want! It also makes enzymes,
hormones, and other important chemicals in the body. Protein is a
building block of muscle, bone, skin, cartilage, and blood.

Of course, there's more to whole food nutrition than just our macros.
The importance of micronutrients cannot be denied.

Micronutrients

We've spoken about macronutrients at length, but now we need to dive into a deeper level. Micronutrients are often forgotten and set aside by other programs, but not here. What are the micronutrients you could be missing out on by not adopting whole food nutrition?

Selenium: this micronutrient does everything from assisting in DNA reproduction, to helping detox your body of dangerous free radicals.

Fluoride: helps keep your teeth white, clean, and strong.

Iodine: is required in order for the body to make thyroid hormones, which affect virtually every system in our body.

Copper: this underestimated essential trace mineral helps build red blood cells, maintain the immune system, and keep our nervous system functioning the way it should.

Niacin: keeps cholesterol levels low and contributes to heart health.

Thiamine: this helps the body use carbohydrates as energy and metabolize glucose.

And so many more, such as vitamins A, C, D, E, K, and all parts of the B vitamins.

Flood your body with those micronutrients. The more berries and veggies you're getting, the better. By consuming more micronutrients, we're preventing cravings and nurturing our body on a deeper level and ensuring our best health.

Which is really what all of us want.

IIFYM

If It Fits Your Macros (IIFYM) is an approach used by some people to eat treats and junk food and still hit your macros (because it will still get *some* results, albeit less effective, considering the quality of food).

At FASTer Way, we use a macros-based approach to fuel our bodies correctly every day with wholesome foods, and we use IIFYM to fit a fun treat in on Saturdays (or whenever you do leg day). Sustainability is one of the main goals at FASTer Way, and using IIFYM to give yourself an occasional treat is one way we create that.

Frequently Asked Questions

Can I adjust my macros while doing FASTer Way?

Yes! We always advocate for you to listen to and honor your body. Working 1:1 with our certified coaches will help you tweak appropriately to what you need. No need to do what isn't working.

Do you recommend multivitamins on FASTer Way to Fat Loss to help me get enough micronutrients?

In regards to supplements, I say have them when you break your fast, and invest in a good probiotic and multivitamin. It's sometimes difficult to get in your micronutrients during your feeding window, and this can help.

How do I know when I should adjust my macros?

If you're seeing results through the FASTer Way with the macros we calculate during prep, leave your macros alone. If you're feeling better, have more energy, your clothes are fitting better, and your health is improving, keep at it! If not, it's a great time to ask yourself some questions, and work with our coaches to tweak for your body needs.

Chapter 6

Carb Cycling

"Prior to finding the FASTer Way, I had been a certified personal trainer for thirteen years. I was convinced I was doing everything right—never skipping breakfast, eating up to six smaller meals throughout the day, and eating mostly protein and fewer carbs. I was in good shape, but still had some unwanted fat around my midsection and thighs. I just accepted the fact that I was now forty years old, and that's the way it would be. I had never tracked what I ate, as I thought that was a bit extreme and I figured it would be too time-consuming. Once I started intermittent fasting, carb cycling, and tracking my macros, I was amazed at how much better I felt even in the first few days. In my first six weeks, I was able to lose my "muffin top" all while increasing my carb intake, exercising less, and allowing my body digestive rest through intermittent fasting."

—*Alicia B*

The Power of Carb Cycling

When I started training clients fifteen years ago, it was the Biggest Loser era—when spending hours on a treadmill or elliptical and eating bird food for lunch was acceptable. As a trainer, I stayed on the straight and narrow by logging my food and counting calories on a daily basis. After all—that was the way to stay slim, energized, and healthy right?

Wrong.

After delivering my second baby, Cole, I continued the 1,200-calorie diet strategy to get my "body back after baby." I was breastfeeding, training clients in the gym for multiple hours per day, leading boot camps, building a house, ramping up my own marketing company, trying to be a good wife, and more.

I was depleted and frustrated, with barely any energy to get through the day. Unsure why I was so exhausted, I tightened up my nutrition and focused on whole foods. As a by-product of eliminating grains, I began a food log with low carbs, moderate protein, and high fat.

One morning I woke up before the crack of dawn, still exhausted, and poured my usual cup of coffee, with the goal of getting at least an hour of work completed before the kiddos woke up. I had web marketing client projects to complete, emails to answer, and online boot camp client check-ins to do.

I woke the kids up and got them ready for the day. Emma was nearly three, and Cole was less than a year old. I ate my typical eggs for breakfast and later enjoyed a second cup of coffee. We had recently moved into our new home Brandon and I built, and I had meetings lined up with our landscaper, pool company, and fence company.

I met with the pool company and discussed the details of our pool install while holding Cole on my hip and trying to entertain Emma any way possible. After the meeting, I quickly drank a protein shake and then welcomed the landscaper to the house to map out a plan. My energy waned. I put Cole and Emma down for a nap and met the fence contractor outside.

A wall of exhaustion soon moved in—big time. I could barely stay focused and keep my eyes open as I negotiated a deal with the fence contractor (coordinating a swap of services like I so often loved to do—I would build him a website if he gave me a discount on the fence install).

Instead of feeling energized and excited about the plan, I struggled to stay upright. I cut the meeting with the contractor short and called Brandon, asking him to come home from work to help with the kids.

I needed to sleep.

I felt so helpless. Me, a personal trainer, couldn't cope with my energy levels. I was supposed to be the picture of perfect health and energy. Yet, I had to call my husband home from work so I could sleep. Ugh.

Desperate to find a solution to the 2:00 wall of exhaustion, I hit the books and started researching. Could poor nutrition be the cause of my tiredness? Although the paleo lifestyle helped me cut down on bloating, I was ultimately becoming more tired over time. I studied each macronutrient and the role it played. I studied carbs, fats, and proteins, which ultimately led me to a strategy called Carb Cycling.

After hours and hours of research, I came upon two life-changing realizations.

God created carbs for us to consume, not eliminate. We need carbs for energy.

I decided to experiment with higher clean carb days through the week, especially on days I trained clients in the gym or did a heavy leg day lift. The results were immediate and amazing. Within days, I became more energized. I eliminated my second cup of coffee and trained harder on strength training days. I had the stamina to thrive through my busy days and energy to play with the kiddos at home. My mood improved, and my hormones balanced out. I still enjoyed the occasional low-carb day but was wise about consuming more sweet potatoes, fruits, veggies, and more.

When I created the FASTer Way, I knew it would involve carb cycling. Carbs are not the enemy. We need carbs, and thousands of my clients have reported a similar experience that mirrors my own.

Low-Carb Diets

Low-carb diets aren't new for anyone.

The first (recorded) low-carb diet happened in 1863, to a portly funeral director named Mr. Banting that had struggled with his weight all his life. After suffering through his excessive weight for many years, he went to his doctor, a man named Dr. Harvey, and asked for help. After successfully losing weight by restricting carbohydrates, he wrote a well-known treatise titled *Letter on Corpulence*.

From its first recorded beginnings in London, low-carb diets have evolved over time. Whether it's Atkins, keto, paleo, or an all-meat diet, we're most familiar with names like *Atkins* and the *South Beach Diet*. But at FASTer Way, carbohydrates aren't the devil. We embrace whole food-based carbohydrates; then use them strategically.

Here's what history doesn't tell you—long-term restriction of carbohydrates and calories can lower your metabolic rate and negatively affect your hormone levels. I see women literally running themselves (and their metabolisms) into the ground doing extreme low-carb diets. This is a big reason why women find themselves at a weight loss plateau. For a short period of time, a significantly restrictive diet will bring you results. However, over time it will cause your metabolic rate to decrease. Once that happens, you will see your weight loss stop and will need to restrict calories or carbs even further to lose more weight, thus lowering your metabolic rate once again. Not only is this a terribly unhealthy way to live, but it is also incredibly frustrating. I am not in the business of making people *more* frustrated.

What Is Carb Cycling?

A carb cycling program is an intentional variation of carbohydrate intake each week. Just as the name suggests, you'll cycle through higher and lower carbohydrate intake. Most carb cycling plans consist of high-carb days and low-carb days. In all of my programs, I base our cycle on the workouts we will be doing to maximize fat burn and energy levels.

In carb cycling, you have lower carb macro days that are paired with higher intensity interval training (and doing intermittent fasting on those days), which has shown impressive results. Beyond impressive.

Sometimes unbelievable.

The beauty here is the seven-day cycle we use at the FASTer Way. Carb cycling helps us:

- Balance hormones
- Maintain energy
- Build muscle

If you aren't eating enough food, you won't build enough muscle, which means your metabolism won't be where it could be, and you may gain fat back. Our metabolism is higher when we have more muscle, which is why strength training is so important. More on this later.

We're very intentional with our carb cycling. We practice it two days per week for women and three days per week for men. We don't do more than this because carbs are the body's main fuel source. We are designed to run primarily on carbohydrates, and if we deprive our bodies long-term, it can start to have a negative effect on our processes.

Men have three low-carb days in the weekly cycle because their hormones aren't affected in the same way as women's. If women have too many low-carb days, this can throw their hormones out of balance, causing more problems.

Carb cycling allows for planned high-carb days that increase thyroid output and help control hunger. Because we're cycling carbs, we also have low-carb days that offset our high-carb days. With this type of cycle, fat loss, increased energy levels, and improvements to our body composition are a constant.

Carb cycling isn't a diet, but an intentional variation of carbohydrate intake. While carbohydrates are needed, it is important that they are timed appropriately to maximize fat burning. The combination of sprint workouts with low-carb days depletes the body's glycogen stores and burns fat, without encouraging fat storage on regular calorie days. Eating carbohydrates that come from fruits and veggies, as opposed to refined sugars and grains, is ideal for optimal energy levels and body composition.

The Science Behind Carb Cycling

Your body naturally stores excess carbohydrates as glycogen and fat, and then breaks them down to fuel your work. Carb cycling mimics this natural cycle and helps encourage the body to break down its fat stores into usable ketone bodies. On low-carb days, you deplete your body's glycogen stores.

Let's say you're on a low-carb day in this program, and you do some high intensity interval training. Thanks to intermittent fasting and low carbs, your glycogen stores naturally decrease. When you work out, you'll have very little sugar in your bloodstream, which causes the body to undergo glycogenolysis to break down glycogen and create cellular energy. By relying on these energy stores, you don't need to eat to fuel your workouts.

Your body will also naturally begin to use its fat stores for energy on low-carb days, too. Once your body adapts to this, you'll feel yourself energized despite its being low-carb day. The combination of carb cycling and intermittent fasting is what really turns your body into a fat-burning furnace.

On high-carb days, your body gets the food it needs to rebuild its energy stores from before. However, because the body first uses glycogen for energy, it will begin to replace its glycogen stores before it stores fat. So, even though you're consuming carbs, your body isn't storing excess carbs as fat because it's busy building glycogen back up.

Combined with the fat-burning effects of intermittent fasting, carb cycling is incredibly effective at helping your body burn fat, even when you're not restricting calories.

FODMAPs

FERMENTABLE
OLIGOSACCHARIDES
DISACCHARIDES
MONOSACCHARIDES
AND
POLYOL

FODMAPs is an acronym that stands for Fermentable Oligosaccharides Disaccharides Monosaccharides And Polyols. FODMAPs are, simply put, sugar alcohols. They're found in foods naturally and as additives. They're poorly absorbed in the small intestine before they pass through to the large intestine.

Two things happen when you consume these:

1) The FODMAPs are fermented by bacteria in the large intestine (which produces gas) and

2) the FODMAPs attract water into the large intestine.

These two processes can cause symptoms such as: gas, abdominal bloating, distension and pain, constipation or diarrhea, or both. If you have eliminated gluten from your diet and still find yourself with the symptoms just listed, try eliminating FODMAP-containing foods, which include (but are not limited to):

Wheat	Garlic	Watermelon
Rye	Legumes	Apples
Barley	Lentils	Pears
Onions	Artichokes	Nectarines
Leeks	Chicory	Plums
Shallots	Dairy products	Cauliflower
Spring onions	Honey	High fructose
(white part)	Mango	corn syrup

Any product sweetened with polyols *(IE—sugar replacements such as erythritol, sorbitol, xylitol, etc.)*

Polyols

Let's talk a little more about polyols.

Polyols are a very popular sugar alternative, so they're added to many processed foods in order to make them healthier. Be sure to read labels! Many people begin to feel better and see results once they eliminate polyols from their diet.

There are six main polyols (also known as sugar alcohols) you should avoid: sorbitol, mannitol, maltitol, xylitol, isomalt, and lactitol. Erythritol is technically considered low FODMAP (because it's relatively well absorbed), but research suggests that erythritol can actually increase the malabsorption of fructose, which in turn could trigger symptoms. Try avoiding it with the other polyols and monitor results.

Low-Carb Days

The goal for our low-carb days is to eat fewer than fifty net grams of carbs for women, and fewer than one hundred net grams of carbs for men or women who are pregnant or breastfeeding.

Men tend to burn off glycogen more quickly (due to differences in hormones) than women and have a higher number of macros to consume per day, thus increasing their net carb total. Many clients choose to eat high fiber, low sugar foods like leafy green veggies to fill up on low-carb days.

Unfortunately, many people tend to undereat on low-carb days. This definitely shouldn't become a habit. Restricting calories can actually depress your metabolism. Undereating on low-carb day and not consuming enough calories can actually be counterproductive. Make sure you're eating enough on low-carb days.

Women tend to come to me saying, "I've been eating 1,200 calories for a long time!" Their metabolisms are bottomed out, their hormones have run ragged, and they've hit the wall. They aren't losing weight, they're hungry, and they have low energy.

Eating enough is the thing that people coming into my program struggle with the most. One of my clients was an Integrative Medicine practitioner that had been eating whole food nutrition for *years*. With that, however, she had been over exercising and not eating enough. After extensive research into FASTer Way, she decided to try it. Once she started eating enough, she was amazed. "Ultimately," she said, "Carbs are okay. It's okay to incorporate good carbs and good fats and what you need."

She still is blown away that she's eating as much as she is, *and* she ended up increasing her amounts later because she knew she needed it.

If you eat enough, you will be happier!

Integrating Carb Cycling

Low-carb days in the FASTer Way lifestyle will likely be the most challenging at first. Remember, we're looking for progress over perfection. Do your best, see what you can improve next time, and keep going. What's more, you won't have to figure it out own your own. Your certified coach and community members will have a lot of ideas and strategies to help keep your carbs low. Your macros may be off, but that's fine for this day. Replace your carbs with fat and keep protein the same.

I KNOW YOU CAN DO THIS.

Frequently Asked Questions

What Are Net Carbs?

Calculating net carbs is simple. Take total carbs, subtract the fiber, and you'll be left with net carbs. Fiber is a kind of carb that is not broken down into individual sugar units and is not absorbed by the small intestine. While some soluble fiber may be absorbed, humans don't have the enzymes necessary to digest most fiber, which means we can't derive calories from it. Because of this, fiber does not significantly affect blood sugar or fat burning and doesn't need to be accounted for in our low-carb gram goals.

Can I have diet soda?

Don't drink diet! Artificial sweeteners (even wine on a consistent basis) is telling your body not to burn fat. I want you to be successful and have a good experience in my program. If there's anything that you feel you're addicted to, we probably need to eliminate it.

Chapter Seven

Workouts

"Before the FASTer Way, I knew that strength training and sprints/HIIT were a better way to burn fat, balance hormones, and become lean and strong. I had come up against a wall where I wasn't able to take my knowledge any further without the help of an expert team of fitness professionals. During the time I've been a part of the FASTer Way, I have gained muscle while simultaneously losing fat. I am learning and implementing strategies for fueling my body with the right macros. My mindset toward my missteps is much more forgiving when I experience less-than-perfect days."

—Rachael F.

The Power of Flexible Workouts

Four short months after I created the FASTer Way to Fat Loss, I was sitting on the beach near our condo with a small group of agency clients and team members on a VIP Weekend. For a couple of years I had been ramping up a small digital marketing agency for female entrepreneurs primarily in the fitness industry, and every quarter or so, I would host a strategy retreat weekend at my condo in Clearwater, Florida.

On this particular day, we were discussing our life dreams and visions. I had asked the gals in attendance where they would live in the future if money were no object. The women spoke of lake properties, homes nestled in the mountains, or mansions with water views.

One of them turned to me and posed the same question. "Amanda, if you could live anywhere, where would you live?"

I immediately looked up and said, "Right here."

One of them smiled and said, "Why don't you move? Isn't your business doing really well? Would Brandon be willing to step down from his job in Ohio and work with you?"

At the time, Brandon worked for Wright-Patterson Air Force Base and had for seven years. He enjoyed a flexible schedule, good salary, and consistent routine. The only way I could know for sure is if I asked him.

I called Brandon right then and there in front of our small group. He answered right as he was getting home from church with the kids.

"Brandon," I quickly blurted out, "What do you think about stepping down from your job, moving to the beach to live in our condo, and working with me?"

Without hesitation—and to my absolute surprise—Brandon immediately said, "Yes. Let's do it."

After I picked my jaw up off the floor, I grinned from ear to ear. "You sure?"

"Yeah. I heard a sermon today about embracing change, and I'm ready."

Brandon quit his job the next day.

We sold all of our possessions in Ohio and drove only our cars and children down to the beach a couple of months later. We simplified our lifestyle and focused on our family of four, while continuing to grow our business. Condo living and the simple life was wonderful and a great change from our routine up north.

The only pain point quickly appeared. We didn't have immediate free access to a gym. We did, however, have access to a park across the street with a running path, a little outdoor training circuit, and the beach.

That's when I was most thankful for the flexibility of the FASTer Way workouts!

On Monday and Tuesday of each week, my client community had settled into a routine of doing sprints or HIIT training. Emma (my five-year-old at the time) and I would hit the beach and do sprints together. (Or rather, I would sprint, and Emma would occasionally bounce along and make sandcastles.)

I could also complete the HIIT workout at home in the condo or even outside at the park. The at-home strength training workouts were easy to complete as well since we used mostly body weight movement and light weights.

The beauty of the FASTer Way workouts for so many clients is the ability to do them anywhere! We have a low-impact, at-home, and gym versions of each workout. And as a bonus, the FASTer Way membership community enjoys live workouts as well.

We Do It Differently Here

When it comes to exercise, FASTer Way does it a little bit differently.

The concept of pairing your food log with effective workouts is what really sets our program apart. We're not just going into the gym, hopping on an elliptical, dinking around with some weights, and going into it without a plan. FASTer Way is a strategic food cycle paired with workouts to maximize results and optimize metabolism.

From its inception, this plan was meant to be sustainable, but particularly the exercise portion of it. I don't have time to go to the gym for hours, and you don't either!

At FASTer Way, we generally incorporate exercise five days per week and rest two days per week, with workout lengths varying depending on the day. Some workouts are only thirty minutes start to finish, and some are closer to forty-five minutes on a heavy lift day (i.e., leg day).

As part of the FASTer Way methodology, we like to lift heavy and do High Intensity Interval Training (HIIT).

Let's talk about why.

> ***An important note about workouts:*** *workouts are important but not vital. If you're coming to the FASTer Way to Fat Loss, and you haven't worked out in years, or you have an underlying issue or an injury that you're nursing, that's fine. I want you to*

focus on nutrition at 120% commitment. We can ease you into workouts when you've healed, or very gradually as fits your needs. If you need to ease into it slowly, move when possible and practical. You can lose fat with nutrition alone.

The Law of Diminishing Return

Compared to fifteen years ago, my clients are doing less exercise overall because there's something called the *Law of Diminishing Return.*

This law states that if you over-exercise or do too much high intensity interval training, you're going to have breakdown. Some breakdown is good—breaking down our muscles is how we build them back up. But this kind of over exercise is not positive. I see this happen in people who are working out really hard six to seven days a week.

That's why my clients are in and out of the gym in 30-45 minutes max. We don't work out every day, but four or five days per week. You can get everything you need done within 20 to 40 minutes. Going over 40 minutes guarantees diminishing returns over time.

At the FASTer Way, you get your day back! You don't have to work out for hours. We strategically optimize our workouts, and then go on with our lives.

Strength Training

We like to lift heavy at FASTer Way.

Our metabolism runs on lean skeletal muscle. That makes it really important to build more so we have faster metabolisms!

Strength training workouts are absolutely critical to building lean muscle, running more efficient metabolisms, and losing fat. Through strength training, we're developing calorie-burning muscle and preventing other issues like osteoporosis.

At FASTer Way, we lift heavy at least two days a week. When we lift heavy, we tear our muscles and rebuild, which makes us stronger. It also increases our metabolism because of our newfound, lean, calorie-burning muscle, which is absolutely key to fat loss. We build more muscle by lifting heaving weights than by doing just cardio.

In my program, long-form cardio is the bottom rung of the exercise ladder.

Throughout the FASTer Way, I only ask my clients to really push themselves when we do our heavy lifting. Of course, it's incredibly important that we don't overexercise when teaching our body to burn fat efficiently, and really pushing ourselves only two out of seven days keeps us in that safe zone.

We often start with working out ten minutes at a time for my low-impact people, and then we move gradually into higher intensity workouts that deplete our glycogen stores so we're burning fat for fuel. Strategic, compound movements keep us away from what I call enterTRAINment, which is when you see someone on Instagram lying on a dirty gym floor using the smith machine wrong because it looks cool on video.

We do very standard compound movements and get a lot of bang for our buck. A lot of that is because we alternate high and low value to maximize results. (I've tested this on a lot of people—and it works.)

On our heavy strength training days, we also eat regular calories and macros. In order to maximize your metabolism long after you work out, it's imperative that you eat the right number of macronutrients to replenish your glycogen stores (in addition to actually building muscles). Which means we need protein for recovery muscle building.

This is where people often miss the mark.

They go to the gym; they lift; they're not sure how many reps, how many sets, and they're not really sure what weights they should use. Even worse—they aren't eating correctly afterward, which means they're unable to see body composition changes.

Without fueling properly pre- or post-workout, those changes just don't happen.

A Strength Training Workout Example

To give you a better glimpse into the FASTer Way program, here's an example of an at-home leg day workout that you can do anywhere.

12 reps x4
Goblet Squat
Plie Squat
Deadlift
Calf Raises (15 reps x4)
Split Squat

Finishers x20
Jump Squat with Cross
Plie Squat with Jump
Star Squat Jump

HIIT

The next element that we incorporate into the FASTer Way to Fat Loss is fasted cardio or metabolic training. This is where we exercise with the right amount of high intensity interval training (HIIT) and Tabata. (Tabata is where we get the heart rate up with twenty seconds of high intensity work, followed by ten seconds of rest, for eight rounds or four minutes.)

Here's a little secret: your body doesn't care how you get your heart rate up and deplete your glycogen stores. Your body just cares that you do. It may not be perfect, and that's fine. Remember: we focus on progress over perfection.

Our HIIT days typically coincide with low-carb days. Our high intensity intervals may include progressive HIIT circuits, sprints, and sprint drill type training. Many times, we incorporate low-impact for people coming in without much experience working out. The whole purpose is getting our heart rate up, depleting our glycogen stores, and burning triglycerides (or fat) for fuel.

A HIIT Workout Example

Dirty Dozen
Complete each move 12 times and repeat the circuit twice
Jump Squat
Skater
Forearm Push up
Curtsey Lunge
Side Lunge to Squat
In & Outs
Dumbbell Thruster
Mountain Climbers
Star Squat Jump
Plank with Row
Toe Taps
Moguls

Treat Yourself—With Leg Day Donuts!

Once a week, we do a heavy strength training leg day. They are our second biggest muscle group (our back is our largest), so we like to work them hard.

Except, after leg day we're going to enjoy a treat.

If you follow FASTer Way on social media, you'll see that we love posting about our favorite treats. Not only do we believe in the occasional treat, but we also make sure to enjoy every last bite!

Frankly, it's a positive thing to have a treat (and to have some carbs) right after a heavy lift. The carbs help to replenish your glycogen stores, and we're going to develop that lean muscle by having some protein as well.

Donuts and leg day have become a favorite amongst FASTer Way clients!

Don't Be Intimidated

Now, when I say *lift heavy* or *high intensity interval training,* I know it can be intimidating, especially if you've never had a structured (but flexible) workout schedule.

Maybe you've watched me on Instagram, and you're not quite sure that heavy lifting is for you. Or HIIT sounds like a bit too much intensity for your tastes. Don't be intimidated. You can do this. We ease you into it because this kind of training is non-negotiable if you want to achieve fat loss.

Here's the deal: I'm gonna meet you where you're at with the workouts.

There's a beginner version of the FASTer Way strength program, as well as an at-home version and a gym version. Additionally, we show modifications of each move during our LIVE community workouts. If you have trouble understanding certain moves, or if you need an effective modification due to an injury, your certified coach will be there to guide you. Your coach and your group mates will also be there to celebrate your workout successes! A workout can seem a lot less intimidating when you have a group of friends who are also participating in the same workout that day.

No matter what, we are committed to helping you be successful, which is why we tailor our programs to what our clients need.

Frequently Asked Questions

Will strength training make me look bulky?

Lifting weights will not make you bulky. Instead, strength training will increase your metabolism and help you look more toned! It takes a lot of strategic effort to be bulky as women, and the FASTer Way to Fat Loss will not cause you to bulk up too much.

How do I know if I have the proper form?

We provide a demonstration of each move in the FASTer Way program portal. We also coach form during our LIVE community workouts. I find it helpful to stand near a mirror at the gym or at-home to watch yourself and check on form.

Do I need a gym membership?

I offer both a gym and at-home workout version. Both are equally effective, and you are welcome to do either.

I have a gym membership (or a personal trainer). Can I continue with them and just use your food cycle?

My honest answer to this question is: if what you were currently doing was working extremely well, you wouldn't be looking into my program. My program is designed to work as a whole. I pair our nutritional cycle with our workouts because that is what gets the very best results. It is absolutely critical that we are fueling our bodies for our workouts and teaching them how to burn fat instead of glucose throughout the day.

Frequently Asked Questions

Do I have to workout at a certain time of day?

This program is meant to be a lifestyle, so just make sure that it works for you. Ideally, if you work out in the morning when you're fasted, that can accelerate fat loss. For example, I usually work out in the morning on leg day, so I am in a totally fasted state. But usually, I work out in the afternoons the rest of the week because it's better for my schedule.

Can I keep doing my normal workouts? (CrossFit, Orangetheory, marathon training, etc.)

Here's the deal. I know that what I present to you is the very best programming in the market, period. I know it's extremely effective. Try my way for a couple of weeks, and see what happens. If it works, keep doing it. Add CrossFit workouts for the social element or for the fun of it on a regular macro day, but don't double up.

I have an injury and can't exercise. Can I still do FASTer Way?

Yes. Exercise is only one part of the FASTer Way, and many people have seen great success with only doing the nutrition aspect. In fact, I've had clients come into the program with a boot on—totally unable to exercise—and still drop eleven pounds.

Chapter Eight

Rest

"At sixty-one, I was tired of trying every weight loss and exercise program. Counting calories was crazy and useless! Feeling run down and frustrated, I signed up with FASTer Way to Fat Loss with an open mind, after seeing another person's results. I felt great during the process. This program is so well put together and is run with such integrity! I finally felt in control of my health! I love FASTer Way so much I look at it as part of the rest of my life."

—Lauren U.

Rest is a very important element of the FASTer Way to Fat Loss. As women, we're going 120 miles per hour every day. When we're overstressed, it's time to pull back or risk causing adrenal fatigue. (More on that in a moment.)

Rest is something I want you to take seriously.

Honoring stress *and* rest, listening to your body, and focusing on whole food nutrition brings about the best results.

The Importance of Rest

There's a reason that rest is the second step in our weight loss pyramid.

Rest is paramount if you want to heal from being sick, particularly if you struggle with thyroid or adrenal issues. Even if you're not sick, or you don't have thyroid problems, rest is still very important to our daily maintenance.

Women, especially, have a tendency to prioritize ourselves last, and that has a detrimental impact on ourselves and our bodies. This is probably the first fat loss program where your trainer is telling you that rest is one of the most important components!

If working out is going to take you a step backward after a stressful day, we don't do it. This is when we bring in rest. If it would be worse for you to go into the gym and grind through, don't do that. We want to encourage listening to our bodies, balancing stress, and honoring rest in our daily lives.

How to Rest

1. Be ruthless with controlling your schedule in a way that sets you up for success. Make important things a priority. I'll let you in on a little secret here: people think I'm insanely busy, but I'm not. I'm just very strategic about who I talk to and when. I don't have meetings in the afternoon, and I go to bed at a decent hour. I'm ruthless with my schedule.
2. Get lots of good sleep. Part of the transition into the FASTer Way mindset is learning to value your sleep.
3. Get outside every day. Fresh air can help ease stress, boost immunity levels, and allow you to mentally recharge[35].
4. If you're starting to feel sick, or you're more tired than usual, that's

when you listen to your body. Feel like you need a day off? Take it.
Listen to your body first, training program second.

5. Get help! I love investing in other people in ways that work for me and my family.

6. Do things that bring you joy. Sleep in a little longer. Go get a pedicure, go to the spa, take time to meditate, or relax in prayer. Whatever feels good and restful to you—do *more* of that.

Active Recovery Workout

On our weekly rest day, I give an option for an active recovery workout—but you don't have to take it.

As part of honoring yourself on rest day, make sure to ask whether the active recovery workout is energizing or draining you. If it's draining you, stop! Do something like going on a walk with your family, take a hike, go for an easy bike ride, or read a book. There's nothing wrong with pulling back. In fact, it's healthier on a rest day to stop than to keep pushing when you just don't feel it.

Undervaluing rest will sabotage your fat loss success. In other words—you need to really take rest days seriously in order to lose fat. At FASTer Way, we're not doing insane workouts six or seven days a week for a reason! Those programs are what caused issues like overuse injuries, hypothyroidism, and adrenal fatigue.

Let's talk more about that now.

Adrenal Fatigue

I actually brought adrenal fatigue upon myself.

Two weeks after my son Cole was born, I started leading in-person boot camps (and had been training for and ran a half marathon while 32.5 weeks pregnant). I was also building a house and ramping up a business. I ended up creating full-blown adrenal fatigue. My body felt like it was falling apart—this is also when I was on antibiotics for sixty-one days because I had strep throat five or six times!

So, if you're experiencing this, I *know* how it feels.

What Is Adrenal Fatigue?

Your adrenal glands produce several hormones, including the stress hormones cortisol and adrenaline. When stressed, your adrenal glands produce these hormones to help your body prepare for intense situations.

During periods of prolonged stress, the adrenal glands stop producing those helpful hormones, which explains the exhausted, fatigued, and fuzzy-headed feeling that signals adrenal fatigue.

Adrenal fatigue is a sign that the chronic stress has gotten to you— and you need to break that cycle.

Symptoms of Adrenal Fatigue

- Wired and tired. In the evening, you're tired, but you can't fall asleep or stay asleep because you feel "wired." You're probably tired the rest of the day
- Your period is off
- Recurrent infections
- Frequently getting sick
- Looking more sickly
- Low workout performance
- Can't get by on six hours of sleep
- Anxiety
- Depression
- Insomnia
- Weight gain
- Joint pain
- Low sex drive

In dealing with adrenal fatigue, keep in mind that lifestyle is a huge factor. Get your rest. Cut back on stress. Don't push harder than you should. If you've had a baby or been pregnant, reach out to your naturopathic doctor. Babies take a lot out of us! Pregnancy, labor, delivery, and breastfeeding alone are really taxing to the body, not to mention the lack of sleep that comes with it.

Frequently Asked Questions

If I have adrenal fatigue, what can I do?

There are adaptogenic herbs that increase your resistance to stress (which means cortisol wouldn't affect you as much without them). They can boost your immunity and provide overall support. Bathing your body in B vitamins is another way to help your body cope through stress. A good sublingual B Complex every single day (methylated already because it makes it more bioavailable for everyone) can go a long way in helping you feel better. As always, talk with your naturopathic or functional medicine doctor for diagnosis and more ideas.

Can I do FASTer Way if I have adrenal fatigue?

Yes, but there are a few suggested modifications that will help you recover faster, such as only fasting 12/12, easing into workouts, and avoiding long-form cardio and high intensity workouts. Also, low-carb lifestyles are known to exacerbate adrenal fatigue, so avoid those.

Can I work out on rest days?

I don't recommend heavy, intense workouts on rest days. Your simple, active recovery workout is fine—as long as you feel up to it, and it energizes you/doesn't deplete you. Not resting contributes to decreased fat loss.

Chapter Nine

Fit Pregnancy and Breastfeeding

"Once I got pregnant with our baby girl, pregnancy cravings snuck in even though I continued to work out regularly. I ended up being borderline for gestational diabetes. On top of that, baby girl was breech, early, and had to be delivered via c-section due to my high blood pressure. Once she arrived, I wanted to get my weight back under control. While I lost the baby weight quickly, the weight that was there prior to pregnancy was not going anywhere with my low-calorie diet. That's when the FASTer Way to Fat Loss found me. This program is pure science. I have never felt more confident in how I feel and how I look. I feel like I can now be a better role model for my daughter. The FWTFL has quite literally changed my life, and I couldn't be more excited to see where it takes me."

—Brooke L.

Fit Pregnancy

Like you, I've long been discouraged by the lack of clear guidance and support for fit mamas. In fact, through my latest pregnancy, I had to visit *three* different providers before finally finding a doctor who was up to date on fit pregnancy research and 100% supportive of my active lifestyle.

Pregnancy fitness has changed a lot in the last couple of decades. Well-meaning doctors, friends, and family members tend to protect pregnant women who are already active and in shape—sometimes too much. We've gone from a really, really conservative place to something a bit more open, but there's still a lot of misinformation out there. Clients often tell me that they know their body is capable of more than the watered-down guidelines most obstetricians will give.

As a personal trainer, nutritionist, and mom of three, I understand how it feels to be frustrated by the fit pregnancy myths, confusion, and misinformation presented online. I care about you and the health of your baby, which is why I created a special program, *Fit Pregnancy*, for expectant mama's. Not only have I tested it myself, but many other pregnant and breastfeeding mamas have thrived through the program.

Because pregnancy can be a very tempestuous time, we've outlined more complex modifications and suggestions to help you through it.

A general rule of thumb while pregnant is to not start anything completely new. If you've been exercising prior to pregnancy, then it's perfectly fine for you to continue during pregnancy. Depending on how far along you are, sprints and speed burst training may be challenging, but you should be able to do modified versions of all strength training workouts—if you've done those types of workouts prior to pregnancy.

The Fit Pregnancy guidelines will also provide nutritional support, with a focus on whole food nutrition, proper hydration, and balanced macros for your body. Although we won't go into the scope of everything here, we also offer a postpartum fitness action plan so you bounce back quickly and never feel alone in the process[36].

Definitely consult your doctor or midwife (even if you have to search around to find one that is up-to-date and supportive!).

Let's go deeper into the FASTer Way pillars and how they apply during pregnancy.

Carb Cycling While Pregnant

During pregnancy, I advocate for you to avoid low-macro days. Your developing baby needs lots of calories to grow and develop! Regular macro days and modified, low-carb days are fine as long as it feels right for you.

Intermittent Fasting While Pregnant

Most women have no trouble with intermittent fasting during pregnancy. However, it is extremely important that you get your calories in every day. If you have to, lengthen the eating window a bit. Undereating has serious consequences even when you aren't pregnant, so they're even greater when you are!

Exercise While Pregnant

If you want guidelines on the best way to maintain your fitness during pregnancy and decrease any delivery complications or risks, the Fit Pregnancy program is your best bet.

The Power of a Supported Body

"As a labor and delivery nurse, I know everything about breastfeeding. Whether it's positioning, food to eat, tricks to employ, the pumping process, or supply and demand, I have it down. I love the breastfeeding connection and helping women find it for themselves.

When I had my daughter, I set the goal to breastfeed for an entire year. Except, I fell significantly short of this goal because I stopped producing milk.

It devastated me. Let me go back to the beginning. Once I delivered my daughter, everyone was talking about getting back into shape and trying to lose weight, so I decided to go for it. My background as a college athlete meant that I always engaged in weight training and volleyball, so I jumped into a really demanding workout schedule six days a week, without a break. I did that for five months straight. I definitely lost the weight, but was totally depleted. And at four months postpartum, I had zero milk supply left.

About a year later, I got pregnant again. Of course, I gained the weight back that I had lost, because that's what happens when you stop working out six days a week! After I had my second, I was back at the same spot. This time, I was determined: I would breastfeed for an entire year.

I felt in my heart that if I knew what macros were right for my body, I would be on my way to a healthier version of myself. It's like the Universe heard me, because that's when my friend Kimmy started talking to me about FASTer Way.

'If you want a program where you're going to eat enough,' she said, 'and you want to know about macros, this is where to do it.'

After my second child, I signed up for FASTer Way to Fat Loss. I was eating way more than I ever have in my entire life—including being a college athlete. My milk supply was insane. I breastfed my second child for almost a full year. (He weaned himself at eleven months, three weeks!) After that, I kept pumping and saving breast milk to give him at night. He never once had to have formula. At one point, I had over 1,000 ounces stored up—which I definitely never had with my daughter!

It's amazing what your body does when it's supported with enough healthy whole foods. Now I'm into my third pregnancy, and I feel totally set up. I still do my FASTer Way workouts five days a week, maintain my eating cycle, and feel better than my first two pregnancies. I have a solid plan going into my breastfeeding journey with my third one."

—Allie J

Postpartum and Breastfeeding

The FASTer Way to Fat Loss is also a fantastic way to get back in shape after having a baby. As I mentioned above, I personally did the FASTer Way Fit Pregnancy program during my third pregnancy with my daughter Lily. My entire breastfeeding journey had ridiculous supply! Some slight modifications for ladies who are postpartum (no low-macro days still, just like in pregnancy), means overall the program is completely doable at any stage of life.

Let me reassure you here:
you're going to see amazing results.

Even if you weren't able to burn fat while breastfeeding in the past, that's going to change. In fact, most of my breastfeeding clients eat more whole foods than ever and *still* drop fat. While breastfeeding my third child, I had an incredible supply through intermittent fasting as well.

Many postpartum moms are understandably concerned about starting the program while breastfeeding. No need for that. Tons of clients come into FASTer Way when they're breastfeeding, and they report a better supply than they ever had before. Why? Because they're eating more whole foods, and they're focusing on hydration. We set your daily calories and macros to a level that is more than sufficient for both you and baby.

And here's the good news—you can still lean out while breastfeeding. A lot of women say to me, "I was never ever able to lose weight while breastfeeding until I did the FASTer Way."

Frequently Asked Questions

How does intermittent fasting affect supply?

Because you are still eating the same number of calories each day, intermittent fasting doesn't have a negative effect on milk supply. Your milk supply is most commonly affected when you restrict your caloric intake. The fasting aspect of the program should not play a role in your milk supply as long as you eat your calories. Keep macros on point and water intake high, as these impact supply.

How does carb cycling affect milk supply?

Since our carb cycle requires you to focus on the specific macronutrients you eat, you'll eat more of the essential nutrients your body needs than when you just track calories. The carb cycle also allows your body to get plenty of each macronutrient without completely cutting one out. This again is eating the way God intended, and fueling both your body and baby's body well!

How does going gluten-free and dairy-free affect supply?

Women in my FASTer Way program do this to varying degrees; however, I highly recommend going through the first six weeks gluten- and dairy-free. Because gluten and dairy are both highly modified during food production, they can be inflammatory for many clients. For those who don't go completely gluten and dairy-free, they typically end up cutting way back on both and still see phenomenal results. Most find this greatly improves their quality of life while having no negative effect on milk supply. In fact, most new moms are told that too much dairy is likely to cause some gas and discomfort for their baby, so this type of lifestyle is truly beneficial for both mom and baby.

What kinds of things should you pay attention to when breastfeeding on the FASTer Way?

Here are a couple of ways to keep an eye on your milk supply: regularly check your baby's weight and rate of wet and dirty diapers. If your baby continues to gain weight and use a normal quantity of diapers, then your supply is doing well. Obviously, if you pump, you will be able to keep a good eye on your milk supply and make adjustments as you see fit.

Part Two

Implementation

So far, we've gone through the structure of the FASTer Way to Fat Loss program. You know what makes it stand apart—the pillars of intermittent fasting, carb cycling, HIIT, strength training, and rest.

While you could try to implement these strategies on your own, I don't recommend it. The truth is this: the true power behind the FASTer Way program is the community. Through community and connecting with other people on the same path as you, you can work through mindset issues, rise together, and achieve far greater success.

We're going to talk more about that in the upcoming chapters.

Chapter Ten

Community

"This community is there when you don't think you need them. They are the ones rooting you on without expecting anything in return. This community of clients, influencers, and coaches is my family. This community is the force to keep going each day!"

—Kelly P.

The Importance of Community

People come to my program for the promise of fat loss, but they stay for community.

I often say there's three things that are needed to be successful long term as you work toward ambitious health and wellness goals:

1.   Intermittent fasting
2.   Eating enough of the right macronutrients and micronutrients
3.   Community

There are studies out there that show that people can live longer when they have strong social ties[37]. When it comes to fat loss and getting into your healthiest body, community is absolutely essential to your success.

If you're not building relationships with people who are supportive and uplifting, you won't be successful in your health and wellness. Happiness isn't about high-carb, low-carb perfection. It's even less about monetary success, or jean size. The happiest people who live the longest have really, really good relationships.

This is why FASTer Way fosters community within my client groups. We encourage each other, uplift each other, and rise together. We create small community groups with a limited number of clients because we don't want anyone to feel like a number. Community managers and certified coaches make sure that everyone has a positive mindset within the group, as well as to encourage and provide accountability and daily support.

Clients are encouraged to share in their small group community each day, and every day they'll receive feedback from their coach. This helps them to stay accountable and motivated throughout the program. It's much easier to stick with new eating and exercise habits when you have people counting on you and celebrating all of your victories.

We're constantly asking ourselves, "How can we be more unified?"

You won't find this anywhere else.

Take it from Denise, who finds power, motivation, and her "people" from the community at FASTer Way.

The Power of Community

"Although I used to oscillate between being a vegetarian and pescatarian, once I hit fifty, my life drastically changed. My mother's warning rang through my mind. 'Once you turn fifty,' she always said, 'you're going to put on weight that you can't get off.'

And I did!

Not only that, but I ended up having horrible issues with GERD and acid reflux. Despite medications, interventions, and time, it just kept getting worse.

My daughter was the first person to introduce me to FASTer Way to Fat Loss. 'Try whole food nutrition, Mom,' she'd say, but I'd brush her off. At the time, I felt miserable on all the drugs they were giving me. I had esophageal spasms so strong that I couldn't speak or swallow, and had to take nitroglycerin to relax the blood vessels.

When my health felt the worst, I scheduled a visit to my gastroenterologist. They recommended that I try no dairy and no gluten.

A light went off.

That's when I realized I was ready for the FASTer Way to Fat Loss. My daughter was excited to have me on board. Within weeks, the dreaded weight my mother warned me about was flying off me. My sleep improved. I even stopped the reflux medication.

That was a year ago.

Despite all the health improvements, the strength of FASTer Way for me is in the people. They are my people! I can turn to them at any time and say, "Hey, can you help me out? This is what's going on."

I drive an hour to and from work every day, so I don't have a lot of in-person friends. The community at FASTer Way totally has my back. I can talk to them about what I'm experiencing, and I know they get it! It's amazing. My husband is the workout guru in our house, so when he's around, I do what he tells me to do. But when he's not around, I love having a community there to help me know what to do next. Even better, I only have to spend thirty minutes working out, and then I can be done. They definitely keep me motivated.

FASTer Way to Fat Loss is the easiest I've had it in my whole life. Not only has it created my people and brought them to me—not to mention they help keep my motivation high—but it's also helped me blast through the issues my mom swore I'd have forever.

I definitely won't now!"

—Denise M.

There's no denying that you're stronger together than apart. While writing this book, I reached out to my coaches in our community and asked them, *"How important has the community been?"*

Here are a few responses:

"Having people to keep you accountable and catch you when you fall has been everything to me."

"The women in this community cheer for each other and truly want to elevate."

"It's been life changing. I thought any chance of getting back to feeling like my old self was gone."

"For me, I love having a community of men and women who are trying to live their best life. I need the accountability and the support."

"The community is everything. I am surrounded by hundreds of like-minded people who push me to be my best and inspire me daily. I have made some life-long friends, and I'm forever grateful."

"It's a huge support, a wealth of information and sharing!"

Chapter Eleven

Mindset

"I found the FASTer Way after losing eight pounds on my own, but really struggled with having a positive mindset with myself and not fully understanding how to fuel my body properly. I would go many days actually feeling starved and angry because I was under eating daily and depriving myself. The FASTer Way saved me. I slowly learned how to change my mindset to be more beneficial and healthy for me. The FASTer Way to Fat Loss has given me my life back in so many ways. Not just physically and mentally, but it's given my family the opportunity to give back more, provide in ways we couldn't, and has enabled me to set big goals for the future. This is the best program ever."

—Jennifer D.

We are often so tempted to count our defeats instead of our wins, but that doesn't help us at all. Part of success with the FASTer Way is learning how to switch your mindset. This revolves around switching from all the negative thoughts that constantly surround us and moving into a more positive space. We do that through having you recount all your victories—and not stepping on the scale.

The Power of Non-Scale Victories

"There are two big reasons why the FASTer Way to Fat Loss has changed my life, and they both exploded onto the scene at the same time.

I have six children—three biological and three adopted. In fact, we dropped right into adopting after having my third biological child and ended up with three adopted children within the year. The hormonal imbalance of just having a baby led right into the high-stress situation of many children.

As a result, I let myself go.

I didn't care about nutrition or what I ate. My skin broke out. My hair fell out. I had no energy and felt depressed. I struggled to get by, didn't focus on what I put into my body, and all the time I spent in the gym only left me more tired. I gave it all up to my family. Until then, I had been an in-shape, fit, healthy mom; I found myself turning into someone who said 'I don't care anymore.' I felt like my body had given up on me. I didn't think I'd ever have the energy and stamina I needed to raise six kids.

A year after I gave up, I went to a rejuvenation clinic. The doctor there drew blood hormone panels. Turned out— my hormones were completely out of whack.

My testosterone was almost negative, my estrogen was sky high, and my thyroid off. They immediately put me on injectable hormone therapy. I gave myself shots every night in the stomach and the butt for eighteen months. Eighteen months and still . . . nothing helped! We saw only a very slight rise in my hormone levels over time, but nothing that we could label a success, so the injections continued. Because of my age, these medicines weren't *covered by insurance. $850 per month down the drain on injectable hormone therapy.*

Finally, in October of 2018, I quit (and didn't tell my doctor). The holidays were creeping in, which meant higher stress. This time, more problems popped up, and I was diagnosed with Ulcerative Colitis—thanks to four ER visits in two weeks.

At this point, I felt totally at a loss.

My doctor told me to go on a bland food diet—basically what you would give a child with diarrhea. They said to stay off of things with nuts, seeds, or anything high in fiber. I couldn't even eat vegetables.

I messed with such a horrible diet for a few weeks, did a ton of research, and finally reached out to some friends with Crohn's disease. My girlfriend in Kentucky had mentioned FASTer Way to Fat Loss a year earlier, but I blew her off at the time. This time she said, 'Look at this program. I believe it will heal your gut and balance your hormones.'

At that point, I had nothing to lose. I said, 'You're right. What else could possibly happen?'

I started FASTer Way in November 2018. Within two weeks I was 100% symptom-free from Ulcerative Colitis and was feeling fantastic. I had more energy, slept better, and my gut was healing. I was able to digest food—I was even losing weight, which isn't even why I did it!

Three months on the FASTer Way lifestyle later, I went back to the original doctor's office (who was still unaware that I had stopped hormone therapy). He said that my hormones were 100% in balance.

'The injections finally worked,' he said.

'Actually,' I replied, 'I'm doing FASTer Way.' Then I explained carb cycling, whole food nutrition, and intermittent fasting.

Without FASTer Way, I would still be on countless, expensive medications, a strict, bland, unhealthy feeding cycle, and unregulated hormones.

My biggest win out of all of this is all that better health has given me—off the scale. I can function, feel good, and raise my family of six kids. The way that my body looks (with less weight) is a mere side effect. I'm seeing this healthier lifestyle translate and flow to my teenager daughters. Their thought processes are shifting into making wise and healthy choices. My son's eczema went away overnight when we pulled him off dairy.

FASTer Way is all about helping other people to make changes in their lives. The main thing it's given me is the health and wellness and how good I feel.

Without FASTer Way, I wouldn't have any of those beautiful Non-Scale Victories."

—Andrea S.

The Scale

At the beginning of every new round of the FASTer Way, I always ask the participants, "Please do not hop on the scale after today!" I have them get a starting weight and take pictures (always take pictures! You'll be so happy you did!) and then promise me they won't step back on. It's just not needed.

In fact, we don't even do an end-of-program weigh-in because it's simply not necessary.

Our focus is fat loss, not weight loss, so there's no need to hop on the scale. We don't need the scale. Smash your scale! That number is not important. Recently one woman emailed me and said, "You wouldn't believe my before and after picture, Amanda! I lost eleven inches, and I'm feeling fantastic."

Non-scale victories are all over the place and are my favorite kind of victory to celebrate and use to cultivate a happier mindset. Because when we celebrate our victories, we inevitably start to talk through non-scale victories like increased energy, better sleep, increased confidence, and anything else amazing that happens because of your lifestyle changes.

One of my male clients dropped his cholesterol by 25 points in one round. A definite victory. Marcia is fifty-two years old and a coach at the FASTer Way to Fat Loss—and a fantastic example of non-scale victories. "My sleeping is better," she says. "I'm filling out and looking healthier. I was tired and depressive while doing intensive Crossfit. Honestly, I never used to think about food before, and now I do."

Because of non-scale victories, my clients are more optimistic. They feel more progress, more passion in their goals, and more happiness.

In fact, sometimes it's uncomfortable.

"I feel like I'm riding my upper limit of happiness and success," some clients say to me. "I'm afraid this can't last, so I keep looking at the negatives." Or I hear, "I don't want other people to be jealous of me, so I'm not going to talk about my wins."

This is why working on our mindset is so important. I want you to experience long-term happiness and move away from that negative space. In fact, I'm going to expect you to constantly switch from negative to positive because this is the final element that makes FASTer Way effective.

Some clients come into FASTer Way and don't drop massive amounts of "weight." One of my clients only lost three pounds in his first round, but his body changed so much that he had to buy new clothes. Then on the second round, the pounds melted off him and continue to do so. If he'd given up after the first round, he would never have known. Instead of focusing on what you didn't do, we focus on what you did. Instead of being hard on yourself because you went over your carbs on low-carb day, or you didn't get all the reps in that you wanted, we're going to switch your mindset to think about your wins. It's all about staying positive.

I call it *progress over perfection*.

Progress Over Perfection

Part of changing the way we think is moving toward a mindset of *progress* toward our goals instead of expecting *perfection*.

My main hope for my clients is that they feel a sense of progress every single week. That may mean they lean out, have more energy, clearer thoughts, greater strength, or feel better overall.

This is why every Monday we have each person set one main goal and then work toward that goal through the week. Setting a lot of goals can be overwhelming. We don't expect people to have ten goals they're trying to juggle—we focus on one at a time. On Friday, I post in the groups asking for wins. Most people have wins based on their goal for that week.

For example, one of my clients had the goal of drinking half her body weight in ounces of water. On Friday, she reported, "I drank more water than I've drunk in years!"

Another person put the goal of, "I want to nail it with eating enough carbs." By Friday, they happily focused on the progress of achieving that goal—even though perfection was nowhere in sight.

We love celebrating those wins together. In fact, we celebrate non-scale victories on a regular basis. I ask my clients to share their biggest non-scale victory of the week within the community so they can inspire others and be celebrated by their group mates. Remember, it's about community.

Also, keep in mind that not all progress has to be physical progress. My clients have seen positive progress in the following ways through the FASTer Way to Fat Loss:

- Eliminating mindless snacking
- Eating their full recommendations of carbohydrates
- Eating enough
- Drinking more water
- Cutting out dairy
- Cutting out gluten
- Waking up without feeling tired
- Less anxiety
- Less stress
- Better sleep

But we've got to come to this program with the right mindset.

Don't come at it with the mindset of defeat right away. If you're saying to yourself, *I can't have those kinds of results. I'm just going to ask for a refund.* Or, *there's no way I can do fasting or workouts like she prescribes.* That's not the right mindset.

Be ready to say, "I'm going to make a change. I want to be the very best version of myself possible so that I can make a massive positive impact in the world."

That's what the FASTer Way can help you do.

Chapter Twelve

Special Considerations

"Living the FASTer Way helped me discover a health issue I didn't know I had. Because I was eating whole, clean foods and working out properly, I knew something was wrong when I suddenly started to put on weight. Within a few short months, my abdomen was bloated every night, and I gained fifteen pounds without changing anything. Had I not been living the FASTer Way, I would have thought the sudden weight gain meant I needed to eat fewer calories (1200 a day) and exercise more. A recipe for disaster for thyroid and adrenal problems. My small intestine bacterial overgrowth would have continued to get worse. I am grateful for the health and energy the FASTer Way to Fat Loss has given me."

—Tami B.

FASTer Way is customized to all people and all bodies, which means we work with everyone. Unfortunately, some of us have special considerations that we have to take into account when working toward our healthiest body. In this chapter, I'm listing some of them here and how the FASTer Way methodology applies.

If you have to make some modifications, do so. FASTer Way can get you to a healthier place faster than without it. Sometimes, it's simply a matter of tweaking the way you do the program to fit your needs. For example, one of my coaches worked with two ladies who were insulin resistant. They figured out they had issues with carbs. After working with the coach to adjust their percentages, they figured out what worked for them.

If you have any questions or concerns, always consult your doctor. For more help, don't be afraid to reach out to any FASTer Way coach that can help customize a plan for you.

Special Considerations

Adrenal Fatigue

If you suspect you have adrenal fatigue before starting FASTer Way, it's important to get tested through a naturopath or functional medicine doctor. It's very trendy to immediately assume you have adrenal fatigue when, really, you just need to exercise more consistently and clean up your diet. Don't self-diagnose and throw supplements at it right away—you want to know your levels first! Then modify the FASTer Way slightly with no more than a twelve hour fast as a starting point, scaling back on intense workouts, and getting lots of rest.

Celiac Disease

Celiac disease is an autoimmune disorder where the body views gluten as an "invader." The immune system attacks the gluten and the body. Celiac disease is a growing concern—many people suffering from this autoimmune disorder are currently undiagnosed. A gluten-free lifestyle is critical for long-term health and success. People with celiac can definitely use the FASTer Way. I recently worked with a local client who saw immediate success in the FASTer Way when she focused on our list of approved foods through the first few weeks. She slowly incorporated wheat and dairy back into her diet and then hit a plateau.

I recommended she visit my functional medicine doctor, who ran a series of tests and found out my client had Celiac disease. Thankfully, we were able to make adjustments so she could continue to see results and thrive through the FASTer Way.

Diabetes

If you have type 1 or type 2 diabetes, consult with your doctor before starting FASTer Way. There is a wide range of varying details as far as fasting and carbs are concerned, and it will be very individualized to each person. If you have prediabetes, you can usually do the program and see great results, but still see your doctor before you make any changes to your diet. Speak with your doctor, especially about low-carb day. Don't participate in the 24-hour fast. Get your doctor's approval before starting intermittent fasting. If given, I suggest starting with a 12/12 intermittent fasting window and working up to 16/8. If you feel dizzy/faint/fatigued after a workout, be sure to eat something.

Fertility

There's a joke that runs through my clients—if you want to get pregnant, come to the FASTer Way to Fertility! While we can't guarantee it, women who are hoping to conceive tend to thrive through the FASTer Way. In fact, we have several hundred FASTer Way babies to prove it.

Gallstones

If you suffer from gallstones, you can still participate in FASTer Way. Because gallstones can cause a great deal of pain and are often aggravated by high fat consumption, low-carb days may need to be adjusted to reduce fat intake. Fasting may also need to be modified, especially if you have a sluggish gallbladder, as it increases the breakdown of fats in the body. There is not a general recommendation for daily fat gram consumption—reduce fat intake enough to alleviate symptoms—but try a probiotic and digestive enzymes to support better digestive health. The same recommendations apply if you've had your gallbladder removed.

Gastric Sleeve/Pouch

People with a gastric sleeve can still participate in the FASTer Way, but be very careful and more aware of your macros. Protein consumption will likely be a challenge, so supplementation will probably be necessary. Always follow your doctor-recommended supplement protocol. Usually, probiotic and BCAA supplementation is acceptable. Be sure to stay hydrated when fasting, don't graze when eating, and don't drink while eating or for an hour afterward.

Gastroesophageal Reflux Disease (GERD)

GERD (also known as acid reflux) can cause heartburn or acid indigestion, and is common in pregnant women. Fasting can aggravate GERD, as stomach acid can build when food is not present, so you may need to modify your fast by increasing the eating window. Otherwise, if you struggle with acid reflux, you can still participate in FASTer Way.

Gluten Sensitivity

While gluten sensitivity is not as serious as celiac disease, it can cause considerable discomfort. With a sensitivity, you'll experience some kind of adverse effect after consuming gluten—anything from abdominal discomfort to headaches, bloating, constipation, or irritability. Once the gluten consumption stops, these signs typically go away. This is one of the reasons so many people feel significantly better while going through the FASTer Way. They are often unaware of their own food sensitivities until they are in the program. Cutting out gluten helps many people feel more energized and comfortable. While those with Celiac disease cannot eat gluten under any circumstance, those with a gluten sensitivity can incorporate gluten occasionally. This allows for various treats without living in constant discomfort.

Hypothyroid

Believe it or not, this is one of the biggest culprits of not being able to burn fat! Hypothyroidism is another syndrome where hormone imbalances produce big changes in the body. The symptoms are very similar to adrenal fatigue because the body's metabolism slows down. That's why weight gain is a common symptom of hypothyroidism.

People with hypothyroidism also commonly feel cold and tired all the time (again due to a depressed metabolic rate). If you have (or think you have) hypothyroidism, I suggest you go to a naturopathic or functional medicine doctor. They tend to look at broader thyroid lab results and view the thyroid path differently than traditional medicine. If you have untreated hypothyroidism, use a 16/8 fasting schedule. Make sure you eat enough—especially on low-carb days—rest, don't participate in the 24-hour fast, and reduce workout intensity.

Polycystic Ovarian Syndrome (PCOS)

The FASTer Way to Fat Loss has helped many women manage their PCOS, including me. If you struggle with PCOS, you can participate in FASTer Way.

Teenagers

Teenagers can safely participate in the program (with a parent) and with doctor approval. Focus on the whole food aspect of the program and supervised workouts as wanted or needed. Eliminate the intermittent fasting, carb cycling, and macro tracking for teenagers under eighteen years old.

Undereating

When we're working toward ambitious wellness goals, it is pivotal that we eat enough! Undereating is a serious concern, especially for people with other special health considerations. To see real results long-term, keep hormones healthy and balanced, and burn fat effectively, you must eat enough. This is something that many newcomers to FASTer Way struggle with. Trust me—eat your macros.

Chapter Thirteen

Troubleshooting

Even though we don't give medical advice at FASTer Way, and we always advocate for you to see a trusted doctor, there are things we can work through to figure out why you may not be getting expected results. Lack of progress happens—and it's typically something we can work through. Your coach is always there for you to help troubleshoot, too. We want you to have the best success possible, and sometimes, finding the exact formula that meets your individual needs requires trial and error.

Let's say you've been working hard, but things aren't feeling any better. Here are five questions you can ask yourself:

Have I started this program within the last six to eight weeks?

If so, give it time to work. Women come to me around the six-week mark feeling frustrated—but they're not quite there yet. Body adaptation takes time.

Am I overly stressed or chronically stressed?

This may put strain on your adrenals and thyroid and prevent your body from burning fat.

Am I getting adequate, high-quality sleep every night?

Without rest, we will likely never see the results we could have!

Could there be hormonal issues at play?

Are you pregnant? On your period? Recovering from childbirth? In menopause?

Do you struggle with unhealthy gut flora (Leaky Gut) or toxic overload?

If you suspect this is the case, I suggest talking to your doctor or your naturopathic doctor to remedy this issue.

If you have difficulty sleeping, high levels of stress, gut issues, or some other hormonal problems, you're at risk for any of this holding you back from getting your success. I always advocate for you to see a naturopath or functional medicine doctor, particularly if you suspect hormonal issues, such as adrenal fatigue or hypothyroidism.

And remember—this can take time! Trust in the process. It takes at least six to eight weeks to see a significant change in your body, and twelve weeks for other people to notice it. There's a reason I encourage all clients to join our FASTer Way community long-term. Decreasing the stress in your life and getting more sleep isn't always convenient or easy. I get it! I'm a busy mama with a business to run.

But, if you don't put yourself first, you'll never hit your goals.

Getting Help

Getting diagnosed with hormonal issues in our traditional medical system is a mess. If you have been participating in FASTer Way and not seeing results, go to a naturopathic or functional medicine doctor.

I've experienced the difficulty of being seen by a traditional, Western medical doctor first-hand. Our current medical culture often makes us feel like nothing more than a number in the system (and, as you know, I've had my own issues with medical doctors!), so I know how difficult it can be to be *really* seen, heard, and understood.

To that I say—support yourself.

Find the people that will help you protect your health and do preventative medicine. Don't be afraid to be your strongest advocate.

If you think something is wrong, but you can't get anyone to really listen to you, know that all hope isn't lost. Remember to look at why things are happening! Family doctors may immediately put you on a medication instead of asking about your food habits, your lifestyle, and more. But that doesn't mean you can't figure something out.

Trust me. I've been there!

I've been to doctors who never asked me about my lifestyle but gave me a pill and said I'd take it forever. (Like my blood pressure medication in high school.) There is hope for people who are dealing with these issues and want to make a change. There are natural ways to reverse problems, so don't give up on yourself!

One client told me, "I didn't know that it was unusual to have bloating, stomach pains, and rampant fatigue. When these things continued during my first round in FASTer Way, I decided to go to a local functional medicine doctor. Turned out I had small intestine bacterial overgrowth (SIBO) and was able to start treatment. Because of that, we dove deeper, and found out I had food allergies that I didn't know you could have. My life has totally turned around since then."

Always advocate for yourself. If you're not seeing results, find someone that will help you take the next step to figure out *why*.

Chapter Fourteen

Tying it All Together

Here's the deal: we need to make sure we're focusing on the right things when we approach a sustainable lifestyle change like this.

The fact that this program will help you be more energized so you can fulfill your purpose is something we need to focus on. You'll be a better, more patient, energized, and happy family member. A fantastic coworker. A wonderful friend.

I've seen transformations. I've watched this program literally save lives, save relationships, and positively impact all kinds of people. I know that these transformations are possible for everyone.

This probably feels a bit overwhelming to think through, which is why I've thought through it all for you. I've given you the resources you need through this book, but also on my website.[38] At the back of this book are some recipes to get you started on your whole food nutrition path.

As you can clearly see now, the FASTer Way to Fat Loss Program is the most effective program available. It's holistic and comprehensive: walking you through everything you need to know to effectively burn fat while increasing your energy.

In addition to tremendous fat loss, you can expect to see an increase in energy, less anxiety, more control over your food choices and mood stability, and much more! More than one hundred thousand people have gone through the program and have seen unbelievable results.

You're next!

Are you ready to make a change?

Do you want to burn fat, increase your energy, and feel leaner and stronger than you've ever felt before?

It's your turn.

WELCOME TO THE
FASTER WAY TO FAT LOSS.

FASTer Way to Fat Loss Cookbook and Sample Meal Plan

The dinner recipes you see here were created in partnership with my personal chef, Donna Giamanco-McCain, a Licensed and Insured Personal Chef. All these recipes are gluten and dairy-free.

Approved Foods List

This list is not exhaustive, but it is meant to give you a better idea of where to start. You are welcome to consume other whole foods that come from the ground or have a mother.

Protein

Lentils

Beans

Hemp seeds

Chia seeds

Tofu

Tempeh Edamame

Chicken breast

Gluten-free sausage

Salmon fillets

Ground sirloin

Skinless halibut fillets

Steak

Tuna

Eggs

Fruit

All fruit is approved, but focus on low-glycemic fruits like berries & apples

Vegetables

All vegetables are approved

Miscellaneous

Black coffee

Herbal tea

Kombucha

Water

Kefir

Protein powder

Nuts

Pantry

Sea salt

Ground black pepper

Olive oil

Butter

Apple cider vinegar

Herbs and spices

Lemon juice

Maple syrup

Honey

Herbs

All herbs are approved

Canned Goods

All canned fruits, veggies, and beans are approved

Chicken Recipes

Bourbon Chicken

Ingredients

- ¼ cup coconut aminos
- ¼ cup bourbon
- ¼ cup brown sugar
- 2 tablespoons rice vinegar
- 1 teaspoon fresh ginger, peeled and finely minced
- 2-3 garlic cloves, minced
- 2 teaspoons of coconut oil
- 2 pounds of boneless chicken breasts, cut into bite-sized pieces
- ¼ cup low-sodium chicken broth
- 1 bunch broccoli, cut into florets
- 1 bunch scallions, cut on a bias

Directions

1. Mix together soy sauce, bourbon, brown sugar, rice vinegar, ginger, and garlic in a sauce pot. Bring to boil, and reduce to a glaze (about 15-20 minutes).
2. Heat one teaspoon of coconut oil in nonstick sauté pan (with lid) over medium-high heat.
3. Season chicken pieces with salt and pepper. Sauté chicken until lightly browned and cooked through. Cook chicken in batches, adding oil as needed. Do not overcrowd the pan; otherwise, the chicken will not brown. Once all chicken is cooked, remove from pan and set aside.
4. Add broth and broccoli florets to pan; cover and steam until tender, about 5-7 minutes. Once tender, drain excess liquid from pan.
5. Add cooked chicken to broccoli. Heat until warmed through. Add desired amount of thickened sauce toss to coat chicken and broccoli.
6. Top with sliced scallions.

4 servings
467 calories per serving
40g carbs / 10g fats / 59g protein
36g net carbs

Quinoa Chicken Salad

Ingredients

- 1 cup uncooked tri-colored quinoa, rinsed
- 2 cups low-sodium chicken broth or stock
- ½ cup almond slivers, toasted
- 2 teaspoons grapeseed oil
- pounds chicken tenders, cut into bite-sized pieces
- ½ teaspoon salt
- ¼ teaspoon ground black pepper
- 1 (8-ounce) package cremini mushrooms, quartered
- 1 cup grape tomatoes, halved
- 1 lemon, zested and juiced
- 1 tablespoon balsamic vinegar
- 1 teaspoon Dijon mustard
- 1 clove garlic, finely minced
- 1 teaspoon brown sugar
- ¼ cup grapeseed oil
- 10 fresh basil leaves, chopped
- Salt and fresh black pepper, to taste

Directions

1. Cook quinoa in broth according to package instructions. Set aside, and let cool in a large bowl.
2. Toast almond slivers in a dry sauté pan over medium heat for 2-3 minutes. Watch carefully; they can go from toasted to burned very quickly. Set aside to cool.
3. Cut chicken tenders into bite-sized pieces. Season chicken pieces with salt and pepper.
4. Heat one teaspoon coconut oil in non-stick sauté pan over medium heat.
5. Sauté chicken pieces until lightly browned and cooked through. Cook chicken in batches, adding oil as needed. Do not overcrowd the pan; otherwise, the chicken will not brown.
6. Add cooked chicken to the quinoa bowl.
7. Add the mushrooms to the pan and allow them to release the liquid and brown approximately 10 minutes. Do not overcrowd the pan, or they will not brown. If necessary, brown the mushrooms in batches.

Recipe continued on next page

Directions

8. Add mushrooms to quinoa bowl.
9. Add tomatoes to the pan; cook until wilted and juice evaporates, approximately 3-4 minutes. Add to quinoa bowl.
10. In a medium-sized stainless steel bowl, add the lemon zest and juice, balsamic vinegar, Dijon mustard, garlic, brown sugar, and a pinch of salt and ground black pepper.
    While whisking, slowly drizzle in oil until all the oil is incorporated. Taste, and adjust seasoning accordingly.
11. Add the dressing, chopped basil, and toasted nuts to the quinoa bowl, and toss to coat.
12. Serve at room temperature or chilled.

4 servings
639 calories per serving
38g carbs / 27g fat / 56g protein
32g net carbs

Sicilian Chicken

Ingredients

- 2 thyme sprigs
- 1 rosemary sprig
- 1 bay leaf
- 1 bunch fresh flat-leaf parsley
- 2 pounds of bone-in chicken breasts, deboned
- 2 tablespoons blended olive oil
- 1 onion, diced
- 2 garlic cloves, minced
- 2 celery stalks, chopped
- ½ cup red cooking wine
- ½ cup low-sodium chicken broth
- 1 (28-ounce) can chopped tomatoes
- ½ cup Castelvetrano olives, halved
- ¼ cup capers, drained
- 1 bunch fresh basil, leaves torn or roughly chopped

Directions

1. Make herb bundle: with cooking string, tie thyme sprigs, rosemary sprig, 3-4 parsley stems, and bay leaf into a bundle.
2. Debone chicken breasts. Save bones.
3. Heat two tablespoons of oil in a large nonstick skillet (with lid) over medium-high heat.
4. Season chicken breasts with salt and pepper. Place skin side down in pan, and cook approximately four minutes or until golden. Flip chicken over, and brown the other side approximately three minutes. Set breasts aside.
5. Add bones to pan, and brown on both sides; remove and set aside with chicken breasts.
6. Add onion, garlic, and celery to the pan, and cook until beginning to soften (3-5 minutes).
7. Add the red wine, deglaze pan by scraping up the bits stuck to the bottom of the pan. Reduce the wine by half.
8. Add broth, chopped tomatoes, olives, and capers. Bring to boil, and then reduce to simmer.

Recipe continued on next page

Directions

9. Add bones, cover with lid, and simmer 20 minutes.
10. Uncover, add chicken breasts skin side up, and simmer until chicken is cooked through and sauce slightly thickens, approximately 8-10 minutes. Remove and discard herb bundle and bones.
11. Taste, and adjust seasonings with salt and pepper. If tomatoes are bitter, add ½ teaspoon of sugar to sweeten.
12. Garnish with torn fresh basil leaves and minced parsley.

4 servings
648 calories per serving
23g carbs / 26g fat / 74g protein
14g net carbs

Amanda's Cobb Salad

Ingredients

- 2 hardboiled eggs, quartered
- 1 teaspoon coconut oil
- 2 pounds boneless chicken breast, cut into bite-sized pieces
- 1 pound bacon, cut into lardons
- ½ cup of frozen peas
- 1 large head romaine lettuce or 2 romaine hearts, chopped
- 1 (8-ounce) package of cremini mushrooms, sliced
- 1 cucumber, peeled and sliced
- 1 cup grape or cherry tomatoes, halved
- 1 pint of strawberries, stems removed and quartered
- 1 cup pre-shredded carrots
- 1 avocado, pit removed and sliced

Directions

1. To hard boil eggs: cover eggs with cold water. Bring pot to boil with lid on. Remove from heat, and allow to sit for 25 minutes. Rinse with cool water, peel the shell, and quarter eggs.
2. Season chicken pieces.
3. Heat one teaspoon of oil in a nonstick pan over medium heat. Add one-third of the chicken pieces; cook chicken in batches until lightly browned and cooked through. Do not overcrowd the pan; otherwise, the chicken will not brown. Once cooked, remove chicken and set aside.
4. Cut bacon into narrow strips, and cook in covered sauté pan over medium heat, stirring occasionally, lowering the heat as the bacon starts to crisp. Cook until bacon is crispy, and the fat is rendered, approximately 30-40 minutes. Remove bacon lardons from fat onto paper towels to drain and cool.
5. Cook peas according to package instructions, drain, cool in an ice bath, and set aside to cool.
6. Wash and chop the romaine lettuce, mushrooms, and cucumber.

Recipe continued on next page

4 servings
660 calories per serving
25g carbs / 26g fat / 81g protein
16g net carbs

Directions

7. Cut avocado in half lengthwise, twist to separate, remove pit, make slices in flesh, and scoop out with spoon.
8. Assemble fresh salad ingredients with cooked chicken and bacon.
9. Serve with lime dressing

Amanda's Cobb Salad Lime Dressing

Ingredients

- 4 limes, zested and juiced
- ½ cup grapeseed oil
- 1 ½ teaspoons agave nectar
- Salt and pepper to taste

Directions

1. Blender method: place zest, juice, agave nectar, pinch of salt and pepper into measuring cup. Using an immersion blender, slowly drizzle in oil with machine running until oil is incorporated. Taste, and adjust seasoning accordingly.
2. Whisking method: place zest, juice, agave nectar, pinch of salt and pepper in a stainless steel bowl. While whisking, slowly drizzle in oil until all the oil is incorporated. Taste, and adjust seasoning accordingly.

> **4 servings**
> **268 calories per serving**
> **9g carbs / 27g fats / 0 protein**
> **7g net carbs**

Chicken Piccata with Mushrooms and Artichokes

Ingredients

- 2 lemons, zested and juiced
- 2 tablespoons grapeseed
- 2 pounds chicken cutlets, pounded evenly to ¼-inch thick
- 1 shallot, finely diced
- 1 (8-ounce) package cremini mushrooms, quartered
- 2 garlic cloves, minced
- ½ cup white cooking wine
- 1 cup low-sodium chicken broth or stock
- 2-3 teaspoons rice flour, divided
- 1 (14-ounce) can quartered artichoke hearts, drained
- 1 (3.5-ounce) bottle capers, drained
- Fresh parsley, minced

Directions

1. Zest and juice lemons, and set aside.
2. Pound chicken cutlets to ¼ inch thick. Season chicken cutlets with salt and pepper on both sides.
3. Heat two tablespoons of oil in a large sauté pan over medium heat. Add chicken cutlets and lightly brown—approximately 2 -3 minutes on each side. Do not cook through. Remove chicken from pan and set aside.
4. Add the shallots and garlic to the pan, and cook two minutes.
5. Add the mushrooms to the pan, and allow them to release the liquid and brown. Do not overcrowd the pan, or they will not brown. If necessary, brown the mushrooms in batches.
6. Add wine, and deglaze the pan by scraping up the brown bits in the bottom of pan.
7. Add the broth, zest, and lemon juice to the pan.
8. Bring pan to a simmer, push mushrooms to the side, making a space in the middle of the pan. While whisking, slowly sprinkle in a little (one teaspoon at a time) rice flour into the sauce; let sauce simmer for two minutes to see consistency changes. Continuing to whisk, adding small amounts of rice flour until sauce is slightly thickened or desired consistency is reached.

Recipe continued on next page

Directions

9. Once consistency is reached, add the artichokes, capers, and browned chicken cutlets to the pan; continue to simmer until the chicken is cooked through, approximately five minutes.
10. If sauce becomes too thick, loosen with chicken broth. Taste, and adjust seasoning accordingly. Sauce should taste lemony and briny from the capers. Garnish with minced fresh parsley.

4 servings
379 calories per serving
18g carbs / 13g fats / 50g protein
15g net carbs

Chicken Lettuce Wraps

Ingredients

- 1 head of butter or Boston lettuce
- 2 tablespoons of coconut oil
- 1 small red onion, diced and divided
- 2 garlic cloves, minced
- 2 teaspoons fresh ginger, peeled and minced
- 2 pounds ground chicken
- ¼ cup water chestnuts, minced
- 1 tablespoon each of mint, cilantro and Thai basil (if available), minced
- 2 tablespoons of fish sauce
- 2 limes, zested and juiced
- 1 bunch of scallions, sliced
- 2 fresh jalapenos, sliced
- 1 lime, quartered

Directions

1. Carefully remove lettuce leaves from head, trying not to tear the leaves. Wash leaves, pat dry, and layer in bowl with paper towels. Place bowl in the refrigerator to crisp the leaves until ready to serve.
2. Heat one teaspoon of oil in a nonstick sauté pan over medium heat.
3. Add half of the diced red onion, garlic, and ginger. Cook 2-3 minutes.
4. Add the ground chicken to the pan and cook, breaking it up with a spoon. Cook until no longer pink and cooked through.
5. Add the water chestnuts, remaining diced red onion, herbs, fish sauce, zest, and juice of two limes. Stir together, and simmer 2-3 minutes.
6. Garnish with chopped scallions.
7. Serve in lettuce leaves with sliced jalapeños and lime wedges.

4 servings
455 calories per serving
16g carbs / 32g fat / 42g protein
13 net carbs

Beef Recipes

Spiced Rubbed Filet Mignon

Ingredients

- 2 tablespoons of grapeseed oil, divided
- 3-4 garlic cloves, finely minced
- 1 tablespoon chili powder
- 1 teaspoon onion powder
- 1 teaspoon salt
- ½ teaspoon black pepper
- 1 tablespoon smoked paprika
- 2 tablespoons fresh cilantro, chopped

4 (6-ounce) filet mignons

Directions

1. Preheat oven to 350 degrees.
2. Combine one tablespoon oil, garlic, chili powder, onion powder, salt, pepper, and smoked paprika in a bowl, and rub over filets.
3. Let meat marinate at room temperature for 30 minutes.
4. Heat one tablespoon of oil in cast iron skillet, or other heavy-bottomed, oven-safe skillet, over medium-high heat.
5. Sear filet approximately 3-4 minutes on each side or until browned. Transfer skillet into oven, and roast until desired temperature is reached. Use a meat thermometer to determine temperature desired. *See guide below.

Rare 125 degrees
Medium rare 130 -135 degrees
Medium 135 -145 degrees
Medium well 145-150 degrees
Well done 155 +

4 servings
508 calories per serving
2g carbs / 37g fats / 34g proteins
1g net carbs

Pot Roast with Potatoes & Carrots

Ingredients

- 2.5 – 3lbs beef chuck roast
- 2 teaspoons salt
- 1 teaspoon pepper
- 2 tablespoons grapeseed oil or blended olive/ canola oil
- 2 medium onions, chopped/large dice
- ½ cup red cooking wine
- ½ teaspoon smoked paprika
- 4 garlic cloves, minced
- 6 medium carrots, peeled
- 6 celery stalks
- 4 cups low-sodium beef broth
- 4 small red potatoes, quartered
- 1 bunch flat leaf parsley

NOTE: Choice of cooking vessel.

Directions

1. Preheat oven to 325 degrees.
2. In a large Dutch oven or pressure cooker, heat oil over medium-high heat; add beef and cook, browning beef on all sides (approximately 3-5 minutes on each side). Once beef is browned, remove and set aside.
3. Add one chopped onion to pot. Cook over medium heat until onion begins to soften and brown.
4. Add wine to pot. Deglaze by scraping up the brown bits on the bottom of pan. Reduce the wine by half.
5. Stir in the smoked paprika and minced garlic; cook 1 minute.
6. Chop two carrots and two celery stalks into large chunks, and add them to pot.
7. Add the seared beef and the beef broth.
8. *Dutch Oven Method: bring pot to boil, transfer to oven for approximately 3 to 3 ½ hours or until beef is tender and shreds apart using two forks.
9. *Pressure Cooker Method: attach lid, cook at 15 PSI for one hour with natural release. Check for tenderness, if needed, cook for another 20 minutes at 15 PSI.
10. Once tender, remove beef from pot into a large bowl.
11. Remove cooked vegetables and discard. Spoon off fat from top of sauce, or use fat separator to remove excess fat.

Recipe continued on next page

Directions

12. Bring sauce to a boil; reduce to a hard simmer.
13. Quarter remaining carrots and celery by cutting in half, and then in half again lengthwise.
14. Add quartered carrots and celery, quartered potatoes, and remaining chopped onion to sauce. Simmer until soft, approximately 15-20 minutes. Remove vegetables, and cover to keep warm.
15. While the vegetables cook, shred beef with two forks, removing fat and gristle.
16. Add beef to sauce to reheat.
17. Serve beef with potatoes, carrots, and celery. Garnish with chopped parsley.

> 4 servings
> 687 calories per serving
> 43g carbs / 22g fats / 66g protein
> 34g net carbs

Chopped Steak with Mushroom Gravy

Ingredients

- 3 tablespoons grapeseed oil, divided
- 2 shallots, minced
- 2 pounds lean ground beef
- 2 eggs, beaten
- 2 tablespoons Worcestershire sauce
- 2 garlic cloves, finely minced
- 4 tablespoons parsley
- 1 teaspoon ground dry mustard
- ¼ cup of gluten-free breadcrumbs
- 1 teaspoon salt
- ½ teaspoon ground black pepper
- 1 (8-ounce) package cremini mushrooms, sliced
- 1 large onion, thinly sliced
- 2 teaspoons fresh thyme
- ½ cup red cooking wine
- 2 cups low-sodium beef broth or stock 2-3 teaspoons rice flour

Directions

1. Preheat oven to 350 degrees.
2. Heat one teaspoon of oil in large sauté pan over medium heat. Add shallots, and cook until softened, approximately 2-3 minutes. Set aside and let cool.
3. Combine beef, eggs, Worcestershire sauce, sautéed shallots, garlic, 2 tablespoons parsley, ground dry mustard, breadcrumbs, 1 teaspoon of salt, and ½ teaspoon of pepper in a large bowl. Mix together with hands, and shape into large oval patties.
4. Heat two tablespoons of oil in same large sauté pan over medium-high heat and brown patties approximately 5 minutes on each side. Remove patties from pan to a plate and set aside.
5. Remove excess fat leaving one tablespoon of oil in pan.
6. Add the mushrooms to the pan and allow them to release the liquid, and brown approximately 10 minutes. Do not overcrowd the pan or they will not brown. If necessary, brown the mushrooms in batches. Remove and set aside.

Recipe continued on next page

Directions

7. Add one tablespoon of oil to pan, and add the onions. Cook the onions over medium heat until onions are translucent and softened.
8. Add wine, and deglaze the pan by scraping up the brown bits in the bottom of pan. Reduce the wine by half, add the broth, and bring to a simmer.
9. While whisking, slowly sprinkle in a little (one teaspoon at a time) rice flour into sauce, let sauce simmer for one to two minutes to see consistency changes. Continuing to whisk, add small amounts of rice flour until sauce is slightly thickened or desired consistency is reached.
10. Return beef patties, mushrooms, and thyme to pan, and simmer uncovered until patties are cooked through or until patties reach an internal temperature of 155 degrees.
11. Garnish with minced parsley for a bit of freshness and color.

CHEF'S NOTE: sautéing shallots or onions in oil before adding to ground meats tempers the sharp flavor onions can omit.

> 4 servings
> 490 calories per serving
> 16g carbs / 21g fats / 56g proteins
> 14g net carbs

Mongolian Beef

Ingredients

- 2 pounds sirloin steak, sliced into strips
- 1 broccoli head, cut into florets
- 1 large Vidalia onion, sliced thinly
- 6 tablespoons low-sodium gluten-free tamari
- 2 tablespoons hoisin sauce
- 2 tablespoons dark brown sugar
- 2 teaspoons chili sauce
- 1 teaspoon salt
- ½ teaspoon ground black pepper
- 2 tablespoons grapeseed oil
- 2 garlic cloves, finely minced
- 2 teaspoons ginger, peeled and minced
- 2-3 teaspoons rice flour
- ½ cup low-sodium beef broth
- 4 scallions, sliced on bias

Directions

1. Cut sirloin into narrow strips, and set aside.
2. Cut the broccoli florets into bite-sized pieces, and set aside.
3. Cut the onion ends off, cut in half lengthwise (root to tip), and peel off skin. Lay cut-side down, slice it lengthwise into strips, and set aside.
4. Combine tamari, hoisin, brown sugar, and chili sauce in a large bowl.
5. Heat one tablespoon of oil in wok or large sauté pan over medium-high heat.
6. Season beef strips with salt and pepper, and sauté until browned. Cook beef in batches, adding oil as needed. Do not overcrowd the pan; otherwise, the beef will not brown. Remove beef from pan, and set aside.
7. Add garlic and ginger to pan, and cook for one minute over medium heat.
8. Add onions, and cook until softened, stirring occasionally.
9. Add tamari mixture to the onions, and deglaze the pan scraping up the bits in the bottom of the pan with the spoon.
10. Add the broccoli florets, cover and simmer until broccoli is tender.
11. Bring pan to a simmer, pushing vegetables to the side making a space in the middle of the pan.

Recipe continued on next page

FASTer Way to Fat Loss

Directions

12. While whisking, slowly sprinkle in a little (one teaspoon at a time) rice flour into sauce, let sauce simmer for one to two minutes to see consistency changes. Continue to whisk, adding small amounts of rice flour until sauce is slightly thickened or desired consistency is reached.
13. Add beef back to pan, and heat through.
14. Garnish with scallions. Serve with rice.

4 servings
256 calories per serving
26g carbs / 11g fats / 17g proteins
24g net carbs

Shepherd's Pie

Ingredients

Mashed Potato Topping

- 3 large russet potatoes, peeled and chopped
- 1 small head of cauliflower, cut into florets
- 1 onion, half with root intact and half diced
- 1 bay leaf
- 2 whole cloves
- 2 garlic cloves, peeled
- ½ cup low-fat milk or chicken broth
- 2 tablespoons unsalted butter
- Salt and pepper, to taste
- 2 teaspoons onion powder
- 2 tablespoons parsley, chopped

Ground Beef Mixture

- 2 tablespoons grapeseed oil, divided
- 1 ½ onion, diced
- 2 garlic cloves, minced
- 1 pound lean ground beef
- 1 tablespoon Worcestershire sauce
- 1 tablespoon balsamic vinegar
- 2 cups low-sodium beef broth or stock
- 2 fresh thyme sprigs, minced
- 1 (8-ounce) package cremini mushrooms, quartered 2-3 carrots, peeled and cut into bite size pieces
- 2-3 teaspoons rice flour
- 1 cup frozen peas, thawed
- Salt and pepper, to taste
- Cooking spray

Directions

1. Heat oven to 350 degrees.
2. Peel and cut potatoes into chunks; rinse and place in large pot, and fill with cold water. Cut off cauliflower florets from head and add to potatoes.
3. Cut top off onion, leaving the root intact. Peel the onion, trim off any loose roots, and cut onion in half with root intact. Secure bay leaf to cut side of onion using two whole cloves. Add to pot with potatoes. Add two whole garlic cloves to potato pot.
4. Bring potato pot to a boil, reduce to a simmer, and cook with cracked lid until vegetables are soft, approximately 30 minutes. Drain potatoes and cauliflower well, remove and discard the onion, bay leaf, and whole cloves. Return potatoes, cauliflower, and garlic to pot. Mash potato mixture with

Recipe continued on next page

Directions

butter and milk, or broth, and whip with an electric mixer until fluffy. Taste, and adjust seasoning with salt, pepper, onion powder, and chopped parsley.

5. While the potatoes simmer, heat one tablespoon of oil in large sauté pan over medium-high heat. Add the mushrooms to the pan, and allow them to release the liquid and brown approximately 10 minutes. Do not overcrowd the pan, or they will not brown. If necessary, brown the mushrooms in batches. Remove, and set aside.

6. Add onion and garlic to sauté pan, and cook until softened, approximately 3-5 minutes. Add ground beef to pan, breaking it up with a spoon: cook until no longer pink.

7. Add Worcestershire sauce, balsamic vinegar, mushrooms, carrots, thyme, and broth. Simmer until carrots soften.

8. Make a space in the center of the pan. While whisking, slowly sprinkle in a little (one teaspoon at a time) rice flour into sauce, let sauce simmer for two minutes to see consistency changes. Continuing to whisk and add small amounts of rice flour until sauce slightly thickens or desired consistency is reached.

9. Add peas and cook two minutes.

10. Taste, and adjust seasoning with salt and pepper.

11. Spray casserole dish with the cooking spray. Add the beef mixture to casserole dish. Top beef with potato mixture. Smooth potatoes over the beef, and bake uncovered for 30 minutes or until bubbling. Garnish with minced parsley.

CHEF'S NOTE: to ensure even cooking, always start potatoes in cold water; potatoes should be simmered not boiled to prevent over-cooking the exterior of the potato.

> **4 servings**
> **604 calories per serving**
> **38g carbs / 42g fats / 31g proteins**
> **32g net carbs**

Spaghetti Squash and Meat Sauce

Ingredients

- 2 medium spaghetti squash, cut in half and seeded
- 1 teaspoon salt
- ½ teaspoon ground black pepper
- 2 tablespoons grapeseed oil, divided
- 1 medium onion, diced
- 2 garlic cloves, minced
- 1 pound lean ground beef
- 1 (28-ounce) can crushed tomatoes
- ½ cup red cooking wine
- 2 teaspoons gluten-free Worcestershire Sauce
- 2 cups low-sodium beef broth
- 1 tablespoon sugar
- 2 tablespoons parsley, chopped
- 8-10 fresh basil leaves, chopped
- 1 sprig of rosemary, minced
- 1 bay leaf salt and pepper, to taste

Directions

1. Heat oven to 375 degrees.
2. Cut squash in half lengthwise; scoop out seeds and discard. Season inside squash with salt and pepper, drizzle with two teaspoons of oil. Place flesh-side down on baking sheet, and bake for 45 minutes or until soft when pressed. Remove from oven, and let cool flesh-side up.
3. Heat remaining oil in tall soup pot over medium heat. Add onions and garlic to pot, and cook until onion begins to soften, approximately five minutes.
4. Add ground beef, breaking it up with a spoon. Cook ground beef until it's no longer pink and cooked through.
5. Drain excess fat from ground beef. Add tomatoes, wine, Worcestershire sauce, beef broth, sugar, parsley, basil, rosemary, and bay leaf. Simmer for one hour uncovered, allowing sauce to thicken.
6. Taste, and adjust seasoning with salt and pepper. If tomatoes are bitter, add ½ teaspoon of sugar to sweeten the sauce.
7. Scoop flesh out of squash with fork, separating the strands. Serve squash topped with Bolognese sauce.

> **4 servings**
> **20g carbs / 36g fats / 22g proteins**
> **470 calories per serving**
> **16g net carbs**

FASTer Way to Fat Loss

Pork Recipes

Pork Medallions with Caramelized Onions and Mushrooms

Ingredients

- 2 (1-pound) pork tenderloins
- 4 tablespoons grapeseed oil, divided
- 1 ½ teaspoons salt
- ½ teaspoon ground black pepper
- 2 large onions, thinly sliced
- 1 (8-ounce) package mushrooms, quartered
- 1 bunch of fresh, flat leaf parsley

Directions

1. Cut each pork tenderloin into eight pieces, trimming off excess fat and removing the silver skin.
2. Pound pork pieces with a meat mallet until pieces are ¼ inch thick. Season pork pieces with salt and pepper.
3. Heat two tablespoons of oil in sauté pan over medium heat. Cook pork pieces until browned, approximately three minutes on each side. Remove pork and set aside.
4. To caramelize onions: cut onion in half, place cut-side down, cut off ends, and peel off skin. Place cut-side down, and slice lengthwise into thin strips.
5. Heat one tablespoon of oil in sauté pan over medium heat. Add sliced onions, season with ½ teaspoon of salt, and simmer approximately 45 to 60 minutes stirring frequently, scraping up brown bits in bottom of pan. Adjust the heat to a lower setting, as the onions cook, to prevent burning as the natural sugars are released. Continue to cook until the onions are a deep golden color; remove from pan; cover to keep warm.
6. Heat one tablespoon of oil in sauté pan over medium-high heat.
7. Return pork, onions, and mushrooms to pan to warm.
8. Garnish with minced parsley. Add half the quartered mushrooms, allow mushrooms to release their liquid and brown. Do not overcrowd the pan, or they will not brown.

> **4 servings**
> **399 calories per serving**
> **10g carbs / 19g fats / 47g proteins**
> **4g net carbs**

Apple Bacon Burgers

Ingredients

- 1 pound bacon, cut into lardons
- 3 tablespoons grapeseed oil or reserved bacon fat
- 1 small onion, finely diced
- 1 pound ground pork
- ¼ cup applesauce
- 2 garlic cloves, finely minced
- 1 tablespoon ground fennel seed
- 2 teaspoons smoked paprika
- ½ teaspoon salt
- Fresh ground black pepper, to taste
- 1 ripe tomato, sliced
- 1 head of red leaf lettuce, roughly chopped

Directions

1. Cut bacon into narrow strips. Cook in covered sauté pan on medium heat, stirring occasionally, lowering the heat as the bacon starts to crisp; cook until the fat is rendered and bacon is crispy, approximately 30 to 40 minutes. Remove bacon lardons from fat onto paper towels to drain and cool. Reserve fat if using.
2. Heat one tablespoon of oil in a sauté pan. Add onions, and cook until softened, approximately five minutes. Set aside, and let cool slightly.
3. Combine ground pork, applesauce, and rendered bacon lardons, cooled onions, garlic, fennel, smoked paprika, salt, and fresh ground black pepper in a large bowl. Mix well with hands, and form into four patties.
4. Heat two tablespoons of oil, or reserved bacon fat, in sauté or grill pan over medium-high heat. Cook patties for approximately four minutes on each side or until browned and cooked through.
5. Serve with fresh tomato slices and chopped lettuce leaves.

> 4 servings
> 685 calories per serving
> 6g carbs / 48g fats / 51g proteins
> 4g net carbs

FASTer Way to Fat Loss

Pork Cutlets and Olive Tapenade

Ingredients

- ½ cup marinated mixed olives, pitted
- ¼ cup pepperdews, or roasted red peppers
- 1 tablespoon fresh parsley, chopped
- 1 garlic clove, chopped
- 2 pounds pork cutlets
- 1 teaspoon salt
- ½ teaspoon black pepper
- 2 tablespoons grapeseed oil

Directions

1. In a food processor, combine olives, peppers and garlic clove. Pulse food processor until combined and finely chopped. Taste, and adjust seasoning with salt and pepper. Remove, and set aside.
2. Season pork cutlets with salt and pepper on both sides.
3. Heat two tablespoons of oil in a large sauté pan over medium-high heat. Add pork cutlets. Do not overcrowd the pan, or the meat will not brown. The pork cutlets will easily release from pan when ready. Be patient. Once meat releases from pan, flip over, and sear the other side until cooked through, approximately five minutes on each side.
4. Serve with olive tapenade.

4 servings
328 calories per serving
2g carbs / 25g fats / 46g proteins
2g net carbs

Pasta e Fagioli Soup

Ingredients

- 1 onion, diced
- 2 garlic cloves, minced
- 2 teaspoons fresh oregano, minced
- 1 fresh rosemary sprig, minced
- 2 thyme sprigs, minced
- 1 tablespoon fresh parsley, minced
- 2 carrots, peeled and chopped
- 2 celery stalks, chopped
- 2 or 3 kales leaves, stems removed and chopped
- 1 tablespoon blended olive oil/ canola oil
- 1 pound of ground Italian sausage
- 1 (8-ounce) can chopped tomatoes
- 6 cups low-sodium chicken broth or stock
- 1 cup uncooked small pasta, such as ditalini
- 1 (15-ounce) can garbanzo beans, rinsed
- Pinch of crushed red pepper flakes for garnish

Directions

1. Dice onion. Mince garlic and herbs. Chop carrots, celery, and kale.
2. Heat one tablespoon of oil in a large soup pot over medium-high heat.
3. Add sausage and cook, breaking it up with a spoon until browned and no longer pink.
4. Add onion to sausage; cook two minutes. Add garlic and a pinch of salt and pepper, stirring occasionally. Cook until onions have softened, approximately 3-5 minutes.
5. Add chopped carrots, celery, kale, and minced herbs. Cook until vegetables are beginning to soften, approximately four minutes.
6. Add chopped tomatoes and chicken broth. Bring to a boil, and then reduce to a simmer.
7. Stir in pasta, and simmer until pasta is al dente about 10 minutes.
8. Add beans. Taste, and adjust seasoning accordingly.
9. Garnish with minced parsley and crushed red pepper.

> **4 servings**
> **651 calories per serving**
> **43g carbs / 35g fats / 40g proteins**
> **33g net carbs**

Spiced Pork with Fruit Chutney

Ingredients

Pork

- 2 pork tenderloins
- 2 tablespoons grapeseed oil
- 3 teaspoons ground cumin
- 2 teaspoons chili powder
- 2 teaspoons dried oregano
- 1 teaspoon salt

Fruit Chutney

- 1 small red onion, finely minced
- 2 nectarines, pitted and sliced into sections
- ¼ cup raisins
- 1 tablespoon sherry vinegar
- 1 tablespoon agave nectar
- 1 teaspoon ground dry mustard
- 1 teaspoon lime zest
- Juice from one lime
- ½ cup low-sodium chicken broth or water

Directions

1. Preheat oven to 350 degrees.
2. Remove excess fat and silver skin from pork tenderloins.
3. Combine cumin, chili powder, oregano, and salt in a large bowl. Add pork to bowl, and toss to coat with spice mixture.
4. Heat two tablespoons of oil in large, oven-proof sauté pan over medium-high heat. Add pork tenderloins, and cook, browning all sides of tenderloins. Place sauté pan in oven to finish cooking, approximately 10 minutes or until internal temperature reaches 145 degrees with a meat thermometer.
5. In sauce pot, combine red onion, nectarines, raisins, sherry vinegar, agave nectar, ground dry mustard, lime zest, juice of one lime, and broth. Simmer until fruit is soft and liquid has reduced by half and thickened.
6. Serve chutney with sliced pork tenderloin.

> **4 servings**
> **459 calories per serving**
> **26g carbs / 14g fats / 68g proteins**
> **23g net carbs**

Pork with Spinach and Beet Salad

Ingredients

- 2 tablespoons almond slivers, toasted
- 2 medium beets, roasted
- 1 tablespoon grapeseed oil
- Pinch of salt and ground black pepper
- 2 tablespoons grapeseed oil
- 2 pounds boneless pork chops
- 1 teaspoons salt
- ½ teaspoon pepper
- 1 tablespoon balsamic vinegar

- 1 tablespoon red wine vinegar
- ½ teaspoon Dijon mustard
- 1 small shallot, finely minced
- 2 tablespoons chopped fresh chives
- Pinch of salt and black pepper
- ½ cup grapeseed oil
- 1 (10-ounce) bag baby spinach leaves
- ½ cup orange segments

Directions

1. Heat oven to 350 degrees.
2. Toast almond slivers in a dry sauté pan over medium heat for 2-3 minutes. Watch carefully, they can go from toasted to burned very quickly. Set aside to cool.
3. Wash and trim roots and leaves from beets; pat dry. Place beets, oil and salt and pepper on a large piece of tin foil. Wrap beets loosely with foil, pinching and sealing foil closed. Place foil on baking sheet, and roast for 45-60 minutes until beets are soft. Allow beets to cool, cut off top and any remaining root, and remove skin with a spoon (the skin will slip off easily). Cut beets into quarters, and set aside.
4. Heat two tablespoons of oil in nonstick sauté pan over medium-high heat. Season pork chops with salt and pepper, and cook until browned and cooked through, approximately four minutes on each side.

Recipe continued on next page

Directions

5. To make dressing: in a medium-sized, stainless steel bowl, add balsamic vinegar, red wine vinegar, Dijon mustard, shallot, chives, salt, and black pepper. While whisking, slowly drizzle in olive oil until all the oil is incorporated.
6. Assemble salad with spinach, oranges, beets, and nuts.
7. Serve salad with pork chops.

4 servings
680 calories per serving
20g carbs / 46g fats / 45g proteins
15g net carbs

Seafood Recipes

Mustard Glazed Salmon

Ingredients

- 2 tablespoons Dijon mustard
- 3 tablespoons gluten-free tamari
- 6 tablespoons grapeseed oil, plus 1 teaspoon
- 1 garlic clove, minced
- 4 (6-ounce) sockeye salmon filets

Directions

1. Place mustard, tamari, and minced garlic in a stainless steel bowl. While whisking, slowly drizzle in oil until oil is combined. Add fish filets, and marinate for 30 minutes in the refrigerator.
2. Heat one teaspoon of oil in a nonstick grill pan over medium heat.
3. Grill fish for approximately four minutes or until lightly browned. Flip over, and continue cooking for three more minutes until fish is cooked through and flakes easily.

4 Servings
483 calories per serving
2g carbs / 34g fats / 38g proteins
2g net carbs

Fish Tacos and Guacamole

Ingredients

Tilapia

- 2 limes, zested and juiced
- 1 lemon, zested and juiced
- 2 navel oranges, zested and juiced
- 2 teaspoons coconut oil, divided
- 2 pounds Tilapia filets, cut in half
- 8 (6-inch) corn tortillas
- 1 small head of iceberg lettuce, shredded
- 3 Roma tomatoes, chopped
- Fresh cilantro leaves

Guacamole

- 3 ripe avocados
- 2 tablespoons mayonnaise
- 1 Roma tomato, chopped
- ½ small red onion, diced
- 1 garlic clove, minced
- 2 tablespoons cilantro
- 1 lime, zested and juiced
- Salt and ground black pepper, to taste

Directions

Fish Marinade:

1. Zest and juice two limes, two oranges and one lemon in a bowl.
2. Place fish in fruit juice, and place in refrigerator to marinate for 30 minutes.
3. To make guacamole: cut avocados in half, remove pit, and scoop the flesh into a bowl. Add the zest and juice from half of one lime. Add mayonnaise and minced garlic. Stir together with spoon or rubber spatula until creamy, leaving some avocado lumps.
4. Stir in diced red onion, one diced tomato, chopped cilantro, and a pinch of salt and pepper. Taste. Add more lime juice, salt, or pepper if desired. Place in refrigerator for 30 minutes to allow flavors to develop.
5. Heat one teaspoon of coconut oil in a nonstick grill or sauté pan over medium heat.

Recipe continued on next page

Directions

6. Heat a dry nonstick grill or sauté pan over medium heat. Add tortillas one at a time, and cook until warmed and lightly browned. Remove, and cover to keep warm.
7. Heat one teaspoon of coconut oil in the same pan over medium heat. Add fish pieces, and cook until the fish is cooked through and flakes easily. Cook fish in batches, adding oil as needed. Do not overcrowd the pan; otherwise, the fish will not brown.
8. Serve with guacamole, shredded lettuce, chopped tomatoes, and whole cilantro leaves picked from stems.

4 servings
588 calories per serving
38g carbs / 32g fats / 46g proteins
26 net carbs

Blackened Shrimp Salad

Ingredients

- 2 pounds medium shrimp, peeled, deveined and tail off
- 4 tablespoons of blackening seasoning
- 2 tablespoons grapeseed oil
- 1 head of red leaf lettuce, washed and chopped
- 1 peeled mango, pitted and diced
- 1 small jicama, peeled and sliced
- 1 medium cucumber, peeled and sliced
- ½ cup mandarin orange segments
- 2 tablespoons scallions, sliced on bias

Directions

1. Heat oven to 350 degrees.
2. Place shrimp in a large bowl, drizzle with oil, and sprinkle with blackening seasoning. Toss to coat shrimp with seasoning. Place on sheet pan in single layer, and bake for 10 minutes or until shrimp are pink and curled into a C shape.
3. Wash, pat dry, and chop lettuce into bite-sized pieces.
4. Peel and chop mango. (Mangos have a large, flat-shaped seed in the middle of the fruit.) Place stem-side-up on cutting board with the narrowest side toward you, and cut straight down approximately ½ inch from the stem. Cut down both sides of fruit, and then chop into bite-sized cubes or slices.
5. Peel skin off jicama with vegetable peeler or paring knife. Cut jicama into a large cube shape. Cut cube into ¼-inch slices. Stack slices, and then cut into matchstick-shaped pieces.
6. Peel skin off cucumber with vegetable peeler or paring knife. Cut cucumber into round slices.
7. Assemble salad with fresh ingredients, and top with shrimp. Garnish with scallions. Serve with lime dressing.

> **4 servings**
> **301 calories per serving**
> **24g carbs / 7g fats / 59g proteins**
> **19g net carbs**

Lime Dressing

Ingredients

- 4 limes, zested and juiced
- ½ cup grapeseed oil
- 1 ½ teaspoons agave nectar
- Salt and pepper to taste

Directions

1. Zest and juice limes into a two-cup measuring cup. Add agave nectar. Use immersion blender, and slowly drizzle in oil with machine running. Season with salt and pepper to taste.
2. By hand method: place zest, juice, and agave nectar in bowl. While whisking, slowly drizzle in oil. Season with salt and pepper. Taste, and adjust seasoning accordingly.

4 servings
569 calories per serving
33g carbs / 34g fats / 59g proteins
26g net carbs

Nut-Crusted Grouper

Ingredients

- 1 cup roasted and unsalted cashews
- 4 tablespoons of gluten-free breadcrumbs
- ½ teaspoon allspice
- ½ teaspoon ground cumin
- ¼ teaspoon smoked paprika
- ½ teaspoon salt
- ¼ teaspoon ground black pepper
- 4 tablespoons grapeseed oil
- 4 (6-ounce) grouper filets

Directions

1. Preheat oven to 350 degrees.
2. Place cashews, breadcrumbs, allspice, cumin, smoked paprika, salt, and pepper in food processor. Pulse until finely chopped. Place mixture in bowl.
3. Rub one tablespoon of oil on fish filets. Roll fish in nut mixture, coating fish on both sides.
4. Heat two tablespoons of oil in a nonstick sauté pan over medium heat. Add fish, and lightly brown fish on both sides, approximately three minutes on each side.
5. Spray a sheet pan with cooking spray. Place browned fish filets on sheet pan and bake for 10-15 minutes until fish is cooked through and flakes easily.

4 servings
545 calories per serving
15g carbs / 39g fats / 34g proteins
14g net carbs

Arugula Pesto Cod Fish

Ingredients

Pesto

- 2 cups packed fresh arugula
- 2 garlic cloves, chopped
- ¼ cup pine nuts
- 1 lemon, zested and juiced
- ¼ cup grapeseed oil
- ¼ cup vegan parmesan cheese
- Pinch of salt and ground black pepper

Fish

- Cooking spray
- 2 pounds cod
- 1 teaspoon salt
- ½ teaspoon ground black pepper

Directions

1. Preheat broiler.
2. To Make Pesto: place arugula, garlic cloves, and pine nuts into a food processor. Pulse machine a few times to form a rough chop. Add parmesan, zest, and juice of one lemon. With machine running slowly, add in oil until mixture is smooth. Taste, and adjust seasoning with salt and pepper. Remove pesto from food processor into two small bowls. One for serving with cooked fish, and one for brushing on fish.
3. Spray a sheet pan with cooking spray. Place fish on sheet pan, and season with salt and pepper. Brush pesto onto fish filets. Discard any remaining pesto used to brush on fish to avoid cross-contamination.
4. Place fish under broiler for approximately 8-10 minutes or until fish flakes easily with fork. Watch carefully to prevent pesto from burning. Depending on heat of broiler, the oven rack may need to be lowered to the second rack position to prevent burning.

CHEF'S NOTE: consuming pesto that has come in contact with raw fish could cause food poisoning

4 servings
450 calories per serving
7g carbs / 28g fats / 42g proteins
6g net carbs

Garlicky Scallops with Spinach

Ingredients

- 2 pounds scallops, cleaned
- 1 ½ teaspoons salt
- ½ teaspoon white pepper
- 1 tablespoon grapeseed oil
- 2 large shallots, finely minced
- 3-4 garlic cloves, finely minced
- ½ cup white cooking wine
- 2 cups low-sodium chicken broth or stock
- 1 (15-ounce) can butter beans
- 1 (10-ounce) bag fresh baby spinach
- 6-8 fresh basil leaves, torn

Directions

1. To clean scallops: rinse, and remove the abductor muscle from the side of the scallop. It's a small rectangle shape that sits on the side of the scallop. Gently pull the muscle off the side of the scallop and discard. The abductor muscle is what holds the scallop in the shell.
2. Once cleaned, pat the scallops dry with paper towels. Place scallops on a large plate, and season with salt and pepper.
3. Heat one teaspoon of oil in a nonstick sauté pan over medium heat. Working in batches, place scallops in pan, and cook for two to three minutes on each side until browned. Remove, and place on plate lined with paper towels.
4. Heat one teaspoon of oil in same pan. Add shallots and garlic, and cook for five minutes or until shallots have softened, stirring occasionally.
5. Add wine, and deglaze pan by scraping up the bits in the bottom of the pan. Let the wine reduce by half. Add the broth and beans. Simmer for eight minutes. Add spinach, cover, and let spinach wilt. Stir in wilted spinach.
6. Return scallops to pan to warm.
7. Serve in bowls with broth, beans, and spinach. Garnish with torn basil.

4 servings
445 calories per serving
42g carbs / 5g fats / 59g proteins
33g net carbs

FASTer Way to Fat Loss

Side Dish Recipes

Brussel Sprouts with Pancetta

Ingredients

- 2 (¼-inch) slices pancetta (from deli), diced
- 1 pound fresh Brussels sprouts, cleaned and root trimmed
- 2 garlic cloves, minced
- ¼ cup white cooking wine
- ¼ cup low-sodium chicken broth
- Pinch of salt and pepper

Directions

1. Heat oven to 350 degrees.
2. Dice pancetta into ¼-inch cubes.
3. Heat an ovenproof sauté pan over medium heat. Add pancetta, and cook until crispy and fat is rendered. Remove pancetta from fat onto paper towels to drain and cool. Reserve one tablespoon of pancetta drippings in pan.
4. Wash and trim Brussels sprouts, removing bruised outer leaves and trimming stem on bottom. Cut Brussels in half.
5. Heat sauté pan with pancetta drippings. Add Brussels sprouts and minced garlic. Cook until beginning to brown, approximately five minutes.
6. Add wine, and deglaze pan by scraping up the bits in the bottom of pan. Reduce wine by half, add broth, and place pan in oven for approximately 20-25 minutes or until Brussels sprouts are tender.
7. Remove pan from oven. Toss Brussels sprouts with diced pancetta. Season with salt and pepper to taste.

4 servings
103 calories per serving
13g carbs / 4g fats / 6g proteins
9g net carbs

Roasted Beets

Ingredients

- 3 large fresh beets
- 2 tablespoons grapeseed oil
- ½ teaspoon salt
- ¼ teaspoon ground black pepper

Directions

1. Heat oven to 350 degrees.
2. Wash and trim roots and leaves from beets. Pat dry, and then place beets, oil, and salt and pepper on a large piece of tin foil. Wrap beets loosely with foil, pinching and sealing foil closed.
3. Place foil on sheet pan, and roast for 45-60 minutes until beets are soft. Allow beets to cool, cut off top and any remaining root, and remove skin with a spoon (the skin will slip off easily). Cut beets into quarters.

4 servings
87 calories per serving
6g carbs / 7g fats / 1g protein
4g net carbs

Roasted Carrots

Ingredients

- 2 pounds fresh carrots, peeled
- 1 tablespoon grapeseed oil
- ½ teaspoon salt
- ¼ teaspoon ground black pepper
- 1 tablespoon parsley, minced

Directions

1. Heat oven to 350 degrees.
2. Wash and peel carrots. Cut off both ends on a bias. Cut in half and then in half lengthwise.
3. Place carrots on sheet pan, and toss with oil, salt, and pepper.
4. Turn carrots cut-side down on sheet pan, and roast in the oven for approximately 45 minutes or until cut side is browned and carrots are tender. Garnish with parsley.

4 servings
124 calories per serving
22g carbs / 4g fats / 2g proteins
16g net carbs

About the Author

Amanda Tress is the creator of the FASTer Way to Fat Loss, the premier virtual intermittent fasting fitness and nutrition program. She teaches her clients how to burn fat and live a truly healthy lifestyle through intermittent fasting, carb cycling, macro tracking, whole food nutrition, strategic workouts, community, and positive mindset. As a certified nutrition coach, strength and conditioning coach, and personal trainer, Amanda spent years in the gym working with people who were doing all the "right" things—with only marginal results. Frustrated, she began experimenting with several cutting-edge nutrition strategies. Her clients immediately started to see a change. Amanda spent years fine-tuning these strategies to work together for optimal results. She has since worked with over one hundred thousand clients and is one of the most successful female entrepreneurs in the country.

Acknowledgements

To everyone that helped me get this book into the world, I want to give a sincere *thank you*. The amount of teamwork it requires to write a book is significant, and I am truly grateful for all the help.

A big thank you to all of my FASTer Way to Fat Loss clients, coaches, and influencers —without you there would be no book. I can't wait to keep changing the world with you.

Above all, thanks to my best friend and husband Brandon and our three beautiful children. Thank you for inspiring me.

References

1 "Definition & Facts for Celiac Disease." National Institute of Diabetes and Digestive and Kidney Diseases. June 01, 2016. Accessed April 25, 2019. *https://www.niddk.nih.gov/health-information/digestive-diseases/celiac-disease/definition-facts.*

2 Stimson, Roland H., Alexandra M. Johnstone, Natalie Z M Homer, Deborah J. Wake, Nicholas M. Morton, Ruth Andrew, Gerald E. Lobley, and Brian R. Walker. "Dietary Macronutrient Content Alters Cortisol Metabolism Independently of Body Weight Changes in Obese Men." The Journal of Clinical Endocrinology and Metabolism. September 4, 2007. Accessed April 25, 2019. *https://www.ncbi.nlm.nih.gov/pubmed/17785367.*

3 Ebbeling, Cara B., Janis F. Swain, Henry A. Feldman, William W. Wong, David L. Hachey, Erica Garcia-Lago, and David S. Ludwig. "Effects of Dietary Composition on Energy Expenditure during Weight-loss Maintenance." JAMA. June 27, 2012. Accessed April 25, 2019. *https://www.ncbi.nlm.nih.gov/pubmed/22735432.*

4 Lally, Phillippa, Cornelia H. M. van Jaarsveld, Henry W. W. Potts, and Jane Wardle. 2009. "How Are Habits Formed: Modelling Habit Formation in the Real World." European Journal of Social Psychology. John Wiley & Sons, Ltd. July 16, 2009. *https://onlinelibrary.wiley.com/doi/abs/10.1002/ejsp.674.*

5 Mergenthaler, Philipp, Ute Lindauer, Gerald A. Dienel, and Andreas Meisel. "Sugar for the Brain: The Role of Glucose in Physiological and Pathological Brain Function." Trends in Neurosciences. October 2013. Accessed April 25, 2019. *https://www.ncbi.nlm.nih.gov/pmc/articles/PMC3900881/.*

6 "Social Support, In-Person or Virtual, Is Key to Sustained Behavior Change." 2018. NEJM Catalyst. May 31, 2018. *https://catalyst.nejm.org/social-support-sustained-behavior-change/.*

7 Webber, J., and I. A. Macdonald. "The Cardiovascular, Metabolic and Hormonal Changes Accompanying Acute Starvation in Men and Women." The British Journal of Nutrition. March 1994. Accessed April 25, 2019. *https://www.ncbi.nlm.nih.gov/pubmed/8172872.*

8 Mansell, P. I., and I. A. Macdonald. "The Effect of Starvation on Insulin-induced Glucose Disposal and Thermogensis in Humans." Metabolism Clinical and Experimental. 1990. Accessed April 25, 2019. *https://doi.org/10.1016/0026-0495(90)90009-2.*

9 "Time-Restricted Feeding without Reducing Caloric Intake Prevents Metabolic Diseases in Mice Fed a High-Fat Diet." Cell Metabolism. May 16, 2012. Accessed April 25, 2019. *https://www.sciencedirect.com/science/article/pii/S1550413112001891.*

10   Tatiana Moro, Grant Tinsley, Antonino Bianco, Giuseppe Marcolin, Quirico
      Francesco Pacelli, Giuseppe Battaglia, Antonio Palma, Paulo Gentil, Marco Neri,
      and Antonio Paoli. "Effects of Eight Weeks of Time-restricted Feeding (16/8) on
      Basal Metabolism, Maximal Strength, Body Composition, Inflammation, and
      Cardiovascular Risk Factors in Resistance-trained Males." Journal of Translational
      Medicine. October 13, 2016. Accessed April 25, 2019. *https://translational-
      medicine.biomedcentral.com/articles/10.1186/s12967-016-1044-0.*

11   "Prolonged Fasting Reduces IGF-1/PKA to Promote Hematopoietic-Stem-Cell-
      Based Regeneration and Reverse Immunosuppression." Cell Stem Cell. June 05,
      2014. Accessed April 25, 2019.
      https://www.sciencedirect.com/science/article/pii/S1934590914001519.

12   "Prolonged Fasting Reduces IGF-1/PKA to Promote Hematopoietic-Stem-Cell-
      Based Regeneration and Reverse Immunosuppression." Cell Stem Cell. June 05,
      2014. Accessed April 25, 2019.
      https://www.sciencedirect.com/science/article/pii/S1934590914001519.

13   Carroll, Aaron E. "Sorry, There's Nothing Magical About Breakfast." The New York
      Times. May 23, 2016. Accessed April 16, 2019.
      *https://www.nytimes.com/2016/05/24/upshot/sorry-theres-nothing-magical-
      about-breakfast.html.*

14   Zauner, Schneeweiss, Bruno, Kranz, Alexander, Madl, Ratheiser, Klaus, Kramer,
      Ludwig, Roth, Erich, Schneider, Barbara, Lenz, Kurt, and Christian. "Resting
      Energy Expenditure in Short-term Starvation Is Increased as a Result of an
      Increase in Serum Norepinephrine." OUP Academic. June 01, 2000. Accessed
      April 25, 2019. *https://academic.oup.com/ajcn/article/71/6/1511/4729485.*

15   Heilbronn, Leonie K., Steven R. Smith, Corby K. Martin, Stephen D. Anton, and Eric
      Ravussin. "Alternate-day Fasting in Nonobese Subjects: Effects on Body Weight,
      Body Composition, and Energy Metabolism." The American Journal of Clinical
      Nutrition. January 2005. Accessed April 25, 2019.
      https://www.ncbi.nlm.nih.gov/pubmed/15640462.

16   Trapp EG, Chisholm DJ, Freund J, Boutcher SH. 2008. International Journal of
      Obesity 32:684-691.

17   Halagappa, Veerendra Kumar Madala, Zhihong Guo, Michelle Pearson, Yasuji
      Matsuoka, Roy G Cutler, Frank M Laferla, and Mark P Mattson. 2007. "Intermittent
      Fasting and Caloric Restriction Ameliorate Age-Related Behavioral Deficits in the
      Triple-Transgenic Mouse Model of Alzheimer's Disease." Neurobiology of Disease.
      U.S. National Library of Medicine. April 2007.
      https://www.ncbi.nlm.nih.gov/pubmed/17306982.

18   Johnstone, A. 2015. International Journal of Obesity 39:727-733.

19   Catterson, James H, Mobina Khericha, Miranda C Dyson, Alec J Vincent,
     Rebecca Callard, Steven M Haveron, Arjunan Rajasingam, Mumtaz Ahmad,
     and Linda Partridge. 2018. "Short-Term, Intermittent Fasting Induces Long-
     Lasting Gut Health and TOR-Independent Lifespan Extension." Current
     Biology : CB. Cell Press. June 4, 2018.
     https://www.ncbi.nlm.nih.gov/pmc/articles/PMC5988561/.

20   Johnstone, A. "Fasting for Weight Loss: An Effective Strategy or Latest
     Dieting Trend?" Nature. February 14, 2014. Accessed April 26, 2019.
     *https://www.nature.com/articles/ijo2014214.epdf?no_publisher_access=1&r3_r
     eferer=nature.*

21   Harvie, M. N., M. Pegington, M. P. Mattson, J. Frystyk, B. Dillon, G. Evans, J.
     Cuzick, S. A. Jebb, B. Martin, R. G. Cutler, T. G. Son, S. Maudsley, O. D. Carlson,
     J. M. Egan, A. Flyvbjerg, and A. Howell. "The Effects of Intermittent or
     Continuous Energy Restriction on Weight Loss and Metabolic Disease Risk
     Markers: A Randomized Trial in Young Overweight Women." International
     Journal of Obesity (2005). May 2011. Accessed April 26, 2019.
     https://www.ncbi.nlm.nih.gov/pubmed/20921964.

22   "Impact of Intermittent Fasting on Health and Disease Processes." Ageing
     Research Reviews. October 31, 2016. Accessed April 26, 2019.
     https://www.sciencedirect.com/science/article/pii/S1568163716302513.

23   Alirezaei, Mehrdad, Christopher C. Kemball, Claudia T. Flynn, Malcolm R.
     Wood, J. Lindsay Whitton, and William B. Kiosses. "Short-term Fasting
     Induces Profound Neuronal Autophagy." Autophagy. August 16, 2010.
     Accessed April 26, 2019.
     https://www.ncbi.nlm.nih.gov/pmc/articles/PMC3106288/.

24   Furmli, Suleiman, Rami Elmasry, Megan Ramos, and Jason Fung.
     "Therapeutic Use of Intermittent Fasting for People with Type 2 Diabetes as
     an Alternative to Insulin." BMJ Case Reports. September 18, 2018. Accessed
     April 26, 2019. *https://casereports.bmj.com/content/2018/bcr-2017-221854.*

25   "Caloric Restriction and Intermittent Fasting: Two Potential Diets for
     Successful Brain Aging." Ageing Research Reviews. August 08, 2006.
     Accessed April 26, 2019.
     https://www.sciencedirect.com/science/article/pii/S1568163706000523.

26   "Fasting: Molecular Mechanisms and Clinical Applications." Cell Metabolism.
     January 16, 2014. Accessed April 26, 2019.
     https://www.sciencedirect.com/science/article/pii/S1550413113005032.

27   Ho, K. Y., J. D. Veldhuis, M. L. Johnson, R. Furlanetto, W. S. Evans, K. G. Alberti,
     and M. O. Thorner. "Fasting Enhances Growth Hormone Secretion and
     Amplifies the Complex Rhythms of Growth Hormone Secretion in Man." The
     Journal of Clinical Investigation. April 1988. Accessed April 26, 2019.
     https://www.ncbi.nlm.nih.gov/pmc/articles/PMC329619/.

28   Carlson, Anton J., and Frederick Hoelzel. "Apparent Prolongation of the Life Span
      of Rats by Intermittent Fasting." Journal of Nutrition, October 4, 1945. Accessed
      April 26, 2019.
      https://pdfs.semanticscholar.org/741d/0f554edc649ffe4bfbf059029f93dd1501bf.pdf.

29   Moro, Tatiana, Grant Tinsley, Antonino Bianco, Giuseppe Marcolin, Quirico
      Francesco Pacelli, Giuseppe Battaglia, Antonio Palma, Paulo Gentil, Marco Neri,
      and Antonio Paoli. "Effects of Eight Weeks of Time-restricted Feeding (16/8) on
      Basal Metabolism, Maximal Strength, Body Composition, Inflammation, and
      Cardiovascular Risk Factors in Resistance-trained Males." Journal of Translational
      Medicine. October 13, 2016. Accessed April 26, 2019.
      https://www.ncbi.nlm.nih.gov/pubmed/27737674.

30   Klempel, Monica C., Cynthia M. Kroeger, Surabhi Bhutani, John F. Trepanowski,
      and Krista A. Varady. "Intermittent Fasting Combined with Calorie Restriction Is
      Effective for Weight Loss and Cardio-protection in Obese Women." Nutrition
      Journal. November 21, 2012. Accessed April 26, 2019.
      https://www.ncbi.nlm.nih.gov/pubmed/23171320.

31   Suez, Jotham, Tal Korem, David Zeevi, Gili Zilberman-Schapira, Christoph A.
      Thaiss, Ori Maza, David Israeli, Niv Zmora, Shlomit Gilad, Adina Weinberger, Yael
      Kuperman, Alon Harmelin, Ilana Kolodkin-Gal, Hagit Shapiro, Zamir Halpern,
      Eran Segal, and Eran Elinav. "Artificial Sweeteners Induce Glucose Intolerance by
      Altering the Gut Microbiota." Nature. October 09, 2014. Accessed April 26, 2019.
      https://www.ncbi.nlm.nih.gov/pubmed/25231862.

32   Martin, Bronwen, Michele Pearson, Lisa Kebejian, Erin Golden, Alex Keselman,
      Meredith Bender, Olga Carlson, Josephine Egan, Bruce Ladenheim, Jean-Lud
      Cadet, Kevin G. Becker, William Wood, Kara Duffy, Prabhu Vinayakumar, Stuart
      Maudsley, and Mark P. Mattson. "Sex-dependent Metabolic, Neuroendocrine, and
      Cognitive Responses to Dietary Energy Restriction and Excess." Endocrinology.
      September 2007. Accessed April 26, 2019.
      https://www.ncbi.nlm.nih.gov/pubmed/17569758.

33   Danby, F. William Bill. "Acne, Dairy and Cancer: The 5alpha-P Link." Dermato-
      endocrinology. 2009. Accessed April 26, 2019.
      https://www.ncbi.nlm.nih.gov/pmc/articles/PMC2715202/.

34   Feskanich, Diane, ScD, Walter C. Willett, MD, DrPH,, Meir J. Stampfer, MD, DrPH,,
      and Graham A. Colditz, MD, DrPH,. "Milk, Dietary Calcium, and Bone Fractures in
      Women: A 12-Year Prospective Study." The Journal of Public Health87, no. 6 (June
      1997): 992-97. Accessed April 26, 2019.
      *https://www.ncbi.nlm.nih.gov/pmc/articles/PMC1380936/pdf/amjph00505-
      0106.pdf.*

35   "Are You Still Consuming Dairy?" 2017. Dr. Mark Hyman. July 31, 2017.
      https://drhyman.com/blog/2017/07/27/still-consuming-dairy/.

36   Jiang, Lihong, Barbara Irene Gulanski, Henk M. De Feyter, Stuart A. Weinzimer, Brian Pittman, Elizabeth Guidone, Julia Koretski, Susan Harman, Ismene L. Petrakis, John H. Krystal, and Graeme F. Mason. "Increased Brain Uptake and Oxidation of Acetate in Heavy Drinkers." The Journal of Clinical Investigation. April 01, 2013. Accessed April 26, 2019. *https://www.jci.org/articles/view/65153.*

37   Terés, S., G. Barceló-Coblijn, M. Benet, R. Alvarez, R. Bressani, J. E. Halver, and P. V. Escribá. "Oleic Acid Content Is Responsible for the Reduction in Blood Pressure Induced by Olive Oil." Proceedings of the National Academy of Sciences of the United States of America. September 16, 2008. Accessed April 30, 2019. *https://www.ncbi.nlm.nih.gov/pubmed/18772370/.*

38   "Spend Time in Nature to Reduce Stress and Anxiety." n.d. Www.heart.org. Accessed April 29, 2019. *https://www.heart.org/en/healthy-living/healthy-lifestyle/stress-management/spend-time-in-nature-to-reduce-stress-and-anxiety.*

39   Holt-Lunstad, Julianne, Timothy B. Smith, and J. Bradley Layton. n.d. "Social Relationships and Mortality Risk: A Meta-Analytic Review." PLOS Medicine. Public Library of Science. Accessed April 29, 2019. *https://journals.plos.org/plosmedicine/article?id=10.1371/journal.pmed.1000316*

Other Articles to Consider

Blackman, Marc R., John D. Sorkin, Thomas Münzer, Michele F. Bellantoni, Jan Busby-Whitehead, Thomas E. Stevens, Jocelyn Jayme, Kieran G. O'Connor, Colleen Christmas, Jordan D. Tobin, Kerry J. Stewart, Ernest Cottrell, Carol St Clair, Katharine M. Pabst, and S. Mitchell Harman. "Growth Hormone and Sex Steroid Administration in Healthy Aged Women and Men: A Randomized Controlled Trial." JAMA. November 13, 2002. Accessed April 26, 2019. *https://www.ncbi.nlm.nih.gov/pubmed/12425705.*

Rudman, D., A. G. Feller, H. S. Nagraj, G. A. Gergans, P. Y. Lalitha, A. F. Goldberg, R. A. Schlenker, L. Cohn, I. W. Rudman, and D. E. Mattson. "Effects of Human Growth Hormone in Men over 60 Years Old." The New England Journal of Medicine. July 05, 1990. Accessed April 26, 2019. *https://www.ncbi.nlm.nih.gov/pubmed/2355952.*

Made in the USA
Middletown, DE
23 May 2019